300 Medical Data Interpretation Questions for MRCP

Third edition

300 Medical Data Interpretation Questions for MRCP

Third edition

Nick Sawyer MB BS MRCP
Lecturer in Nephrology, The Renal Unit, The London Hospital, London

Roger Gabriel BA MB MSc FRCP
Renal Physician, St Mary's Hospital, London

Cynthia M. Gabriel MB FRCP DCH
Consultant Paediatrician, St Albans City Hospital, Hertfordshire

Butterworths
London Boston Singapore Sydney Toronto Wellington

🜨 PART OF REED INTERNATIONAL P.L.C.

First published 1978
Reprinted 1979
Second edition 1982
Reprinted 1987
Third edition 1989

Butterworth & Co. (Publishers) Ltd, 1989

British Library Cataloguing in Publication Data

300 medical data interpretation questions for MRCP –
3rd ed.
1. Medicine. Diagnosis. Data. Interpretation
– Questions and answers
I. Title II. Sawyer, Nick III. Gabriel,
Cynthia M. IV. Gabriel, Roger. Medical data
interpretation for MRCP
616.07'5'076

ISBN 0–407–01650–3

Library of Congress Cataloging in Publication Data

Sawyer, Nick.
  300 medical data interpretation questions for MRCP/Nick Sawyer,
Roger Gabriel, Cynthia M. Gabriel. — 3rd ed.
    p. cm.
  Rev. ed. of: Medical data interpretation for MRCP/Roger Gabriel,
Cynthia M. Gabriel. 2nd ed. 1982.
    ISBN 0–407–01650–3 :
    1. Diagnosis—Examinations, questions, etc. 2. Internal medicine—
Examinations, questions, etc. I. Gabriel, Roger. II. Gabriel,
Cynthia M. III. Gabriel, Roger. Medical data interpretation for
MRCP. IV. Title. V. Title: Three hundred medical data interpretation
questions for MRCP.
    [DNLM: 1. Diagnosis—examination questions. WB 18 S271m]
RC71.S188 1989
616.07'5'076—dc19

Laserset by Scribe Design, Gillingham, Kent
Printed and bound in Great Britain by Page Bros Ltd, Norwich, Norfolk

Preface to the third edition

In the MRCP(UK) examination 45 minutes are allotted in which to answer 10 data interpretation questions. In the third edition the questions have been rearranged into 30 papers of 10 questions each, mainly set out in a format similar to that in the examination. There are 50 new questions, 55 deletions and over 175 revisions. Short answers are required in the examination but this book provides amplification and clarification. The questions, like those in the examination, vary from the straightforward to the more complex. This edition also contains a topic index to aid revision.

N.S
R.G
C.M.G
February 1989

Preface to the first edition

Passing the MRCP diploma is the entrance to serious postgraduate training. The sooner this examination has been passed the sooner the doctor can proceed with his career.

Success in examinations is in part familiarity with the kinds of questions set. We have written this book so that the MRCP candidate may practise his approach to the data section of the diploma.

We would like to thank the staff of Butterworths for their patience and assistance in producing this work.

R.G.
C.M.G.

Normal ranges of concentrations of biological substances

The normal range for biochemical and haematological concentrations varies to some extent from laboratory to laboratory. The figures quoted below are those used as normals for the purpose of this book.

BIOCHEMICAL

Plasma or serum	SI units	Conventional units
Acid phosphatase (prostatic)	0–1.0 iu/l	0–0.5 King–Armstrong units/100 ml
Acid phosphatase (total)	0.9–5.4 iu/l	0.5–3.0 King–Armstrong units/100 ml
Alanine transaminase (ALT/SGPT)	5–30 iu/l	
Albumin	39–45 g/l	3.9–4.5 g/100 ml
Aldosterone	100–330 pmol/l	3.5–12 ng/100 ml
Alkaline phosphatase (adults)	21–92 iu/l	3–13 King–Armstrong units/100 ml
Amylase	150–340 iu/l	80–180 Somogyi units/ 100 ml
Aspartate transaminase (AST/SGOT)	5–30 iu/l	
Bicarbonate	22–28 mmol/l	22–28 mEq/l
Bilirubin	3–20 µmol/l	0.1–1.1 mg/100 ml
Ceruloplasmin	1.8–2.5 µmol/l	27–37 mg/dl
Calcium	2.25–2.6 mmol/l	9–10.4 mg/100 ml
Chloride	98–108 mmol/l	98–108 mEq/l
Cholesterol		
young adults	4.1–7.3 mmol/l	160–280 mg/100 ml
elderly	5.2–9.0 mmol/l	200–350 mg/100 ml
C3 (third component of the complement cascade)	0.1–0.18 g/l	100–180 mg/100 ml
Copper	14–22 µmol/l	17–160 µg/100 ml
Cortisol		
09.00 hours	140–700 nmol/l	5.0–25.5 µg/100 ml
24.00 hours	less than 140 nmol/l	less than 5.0 µg/100 ml

Plasma or serum	SI units	Conventional units
Creatine kinase (CPK)		
males	less than 100 iu/l	
females	less than 65 iu/l	
Creatinine		
young adults	53–133 μmol/l	0.6–1.5 mg/100 ml
elderly	70–168 μmol/l	0.8–1.9 mg/100 ml
DNA binding		less than 30%
Ferritin	20–300 μg/l	20–300 ng/ml
Fibrinogen	0.2–0.4 g/l	200–400 mg/100 ml
Globulin	21–36 g/l	2.1–3.6 g/100 ml
Glucose (venous, fasting)	3.6–6.1 mmol/l	65–110 mg/100 ml
Glucose (CSF)	3.3–4.4 mmol/l	60–80 mg/100 ml
γ-Glutamyl transpeptidase		
(γ-GT)	5–30 iu/l	
Immunoglobulin G (IgG)	5–14 g/l	500–1400 mg/100 ml
Immunoglobulin A (IgA)	0.5–3.0 g/l	50–300 mg/100 ml
Immunoglobulin M (IgM)		
(adults)	0.5–2.0 g/l	50–200 mg/100 ml
Iron		
males	8–30 μmol/l	45–168 μg/100 ml
females	4–30 μmol/l	22.5–168 μg/100 ml
Iron binding capacity	45–72 μmol/l	250–400 μg/100 ml
Magnesium	0.7–0.95 mmol/l	2.8–3.8 mg/100 ml
Noradrenaline		
(normotensive, lying,		
Caucasian)		200–600 pg/ml plasma
5-Nucleotidase (5-NT)	4–15 iu/l	
Osmolarity	285–295 mOsm/l	285–295 mOsm/l
P_{CO_2}	4.7–6.0 kPa	35–45 mmHg
P_{O_2}	11.3–14.0 kPa	85–105 mmHg
pH	36–43 nmol/l	7.45–7.36
Phosphate (fasting)	0.7–1.4 mmol/l	2.2–4.3 mg/100 ml
Potassium	3.0–5.5 mmol/l	3.0–5.5 mEq/l
Protein (total)	62–82 g/l	6.2–8.2 g/100 ml
Protein (CSF)	0.15–0.4 g/l	15–40 mg/100 ml
Protein bound iodine	280–630 nmol/l	3.5–8.0 μg/100 ml
Renin (basal, normal sodium		
diet, normotensive)	200–2000 pg ml^{-1} h^{-1}*	
Sodium	135–146 mmol/l	135–146 mEq/l
Thyroxine (T4)	60–140 nmol/l	4.7–10.9 μg/100 ml
Triiodothyroxine (T3)	1.2–3.0 nmol/l	1.85–4.62 ng/ml
Triiodothyronine (T3)		
uptake**		90–117%
Triglycerides (fasting)	0.8–1.7 nmol/l	70–150 mg/100 ml
TSH	1–6 mU/l	1–6 iu/ml
Urate† (uric acid)		
males	0.20–0.39 mmol/l	3.5–6.5 mg/100 ml
females	0.19–0.36 mmol/l	3.0–6.0 mg/100 ml
Urea†	3.3–6.6 mmol/l	20–40 mg/100 ml

*in SI units pg ml^{-1} h^{-1} is equivalent to pg/ml/h
**reduced values indicate hyperthyroidism or hypoproteinaemia
†increase in concentration with increasing age

Urine	SI units	Conventional units
Aldosterone	14–40 nmol/24 h	2–10 μg/24 h
Amylase		up to 3000 Somogyi units/24 hours
Calcium*		
males	2.5–7.5 mmol/24 h	100–300 mg/24 h
females	2.5–6.25 mmol/24 h	100–250 mg/24 h
Copper	15–78 μmol/24 h	5–25 μg/24 h
Creatinine†	9–11 mmol/24 h	1015–1245 mg/24 h
HMMA (VMA) 4-hydroxy-3-methoxy-mandelic acid	10–35 μmol/24 h	2–7 mg/24 h
Metanephrines	0.5–7.0 μmol/24 h	0.09–1.3 mg/24 h
Phosphate*	32–64 mmol/24 h	1000–2000 mg/24 h
Potassium*	30–150 mmol/24 h	30–150 mEq/24 h
Protein	less than 0.2 g/24 h	less than 200 mg/24 h
Sodium*	80–200 mmol/24 h	80–200 mEq/24 h
Urea*	250–600 mmol/24 h	15–36 g/24 h

Cerebrospinal fluid		
Protein	0.15–0.4 g/l	15–40 mg/100 ml
Glucose	>3.5 mmol/l	68 mg/100 ml
	or over 45% of simultaneous blood glucose	

Faeces		
Fat	11–20 mmol/24 h	3–6 g/24 h

*considerable variation with diet
†varies with muscle mass

HAEMATOLOGICAL

Plasma		
Haemoglobin		
males	113–180 g/l	13–18 g/100 ml
females	115–150 g/l	11.5–15 g/100 ml
Red blood cell count		
males	$4.5–6.5 \times 10^{12}$/l	$4.5–6.5 \times 10^{6}$/mm^3
females	$3.9–5.6 \times 10^{12}$/l	$3.9–5.6 \times 10^{6}$/mm^3
Packed-cell volume (PCV)		
males	0.40–0.54	40–54%
females	0.35–0.47	35–47%
Mean corpuscular haemoglobin (MCH)	27–32 pg	27–32 μμg
Mean corpuscular haemoglobin concentration (MCH)	32–36 g/dl	32–36 g/100 ml
Mean corpuscular volume (MCV)	76–100 fl	76–100 μm^3
Platelet count	$150–400 \times 10^{9}$/l	150 000–400 000/mm^3
Reticulocyte count		0.2–2%
White blood cell count (WBC) (total)	$4.0–11.0 \times 10^{9}$/l	4000–11 000/mm^3

Plasma	SI units	Conventional units
Differential WBC		
Neutrophils	$2.5–7.5 \times 10^9/l$	$2500–7500/mm^3$
Lymphocytes	$1.5–3.5 \times 10^9/l$	$1500–3500/mm^3$
Eosinophils	$0.04–0.44 \times 10^9/l$	$40–440/mm^3$
Basophils	$0.0–0.1 \times 10^9/l$	$0–100/mm^3$
Monocytes	$0.2–0.8 \times 10^9/l$	$200–800/mm^3$
Vitamin B_{12}	90–443 pmol/l	120–600 pg/ml
Folate (red cell)	280–1360 nmol/l cells	125–600 ng/ml cells
Folate (serum)	14–140 nmol/l	2.1–21 ng/ml

Index to questions

Paper 1

Question 1.1

The following figures were obtained at cardiac catheterization from an asymptomatic child aged 10 years:

Chamber	Pressure (mmHg)	Oxygen saturation (%)
Superior vena cava	–	69
Inferior vena cava	–	65
Right atrium	10	81
Right ventricle	35/0	80
Pulmonary artery	35/12	80
Left atrium	12	96
Left ventricle	105/0	95
Femoral artery	105/55	95

What was the diagnosis?

Question 1.2

A man aged 29 years developed an acute respiratory illness with fever and cough. Investigations: chest X-rays—right mid-zone consolidation; white blood cell count $4.0 \times 10^9/l$ (4000/mm^3) with a normal differential; attempts to make a blood film failed as erythrocytes agglutinated on the slide; sputum—blood stained, no bacterial pathogens cultured.

(a) What was the probable diagnosis?
(b) Suggest two tests to substantiate the diagnosis.
(c) What is the treatment?

1

Question 1.3

A 50-year-old woman has ascites that is found to contain albumin at a concentration of 21 g/l (2.1 g/100 ml).

State three possible diagnoses

Question 1.4

A man aged 57 years had an emergency partial gastrectomy. The next day he was found to have a urine flow of 15 ml per hour. Investigations: electrolytes normal; blood urea 16 mmol/l (100 mg/100 ml); serum osmolarity 295 mmol/l; urine osmolarity 700 mmol/l; urine sodium 23 mmol/l (mEq/l).

Was this: dehydration; over-hydration; or acute renal failure?

Question 1.5

A 35-year-old woman has a history of tripping over her right foot and intermittent blurred vision for 9 months. CSF under normal pressure contained the following: 1 cell/2 hpf; glucose 4.3 mmol/1 (77.5 mg/100 ml), blood glucose taken at the same time 6.4 mmol/l (115 mg/100 ml); total protein 0.4 g/l (40 mg/100 ml); electrophoresis of CSF protein showed that the gamma globulin content was twice normal; VDRL/TPHA negative; colloidal gold curve—first-zone abnormality.

(*a*) What diagnosis was likely?
(*b*) What other specific abnormalities might have been found in the CSF?

Question 1.6

A woman aged 62 years had persistent vomiting. Investigations: barium meal normal; blood urea 29 mmol/l (175 mg/100 ml); serum calcium 3.8 mmol/l (13.5 mg/100 ml); serum phosphate 1.8 mmol/l (5.5 mg/100 ml); alkaline phosphatase 71 iu/l (10 King–Armstrong units/100 ml); serum albumin 40 g/l (4.0 g/100 ml); Hb 9.7 g/dl (g/100 ml).

(*a*) What was the cause of the vomiting?
(*b*) Suggest two diagnoses.

Question 1.7

An ill woman aged 59 years was found to have a serum iron of 10 μmol/l (56 μg/100 ml) in blood sampled at 16.00 hours. Plasma ferritin 200 μg/l.

(a) What is the explanation of these findings?
(b) What further tests may be required?

Question 1.8

A woman aged 27 years had a bitemporal headache and was found to have a diastolic blood pressure of 105 mmHg. Investigations: plasma potassium 3.1 mmol/l (mEq/l); serum cortisol measured at 09.00 hours 990 nmol/l (35.8 μg/100 ml). She was given dexamethasone 8 mg daily. On day 2 serum cortisol was 340 nmol/l (12.3 μg/100 ml) and on day 3 sampled at the same time serum cortisol was 130 nmol/l (4.7 μg/100 ml).

(a) What was the diagnosis?
(b) How may the condition be treated?

Question 1.9

A boy aged 4 years suffered from eczema and had a history of infections and bruising. Investigations: Hb 8.5 g/dl (g/100 ml); platelet count 70 $\times$ 10^9/l (70 000/mm^3); serum IgM 0.3 g/l (300 mg/100 ml); IgA 3.8 g/l (3800 mg/100 ml); IgG 4.7 g/l (4700 mg/100 ml); T-cell count 172 $\times$ 10^3/l; B-cell count 343 $\times$ 10^3/l.

(a) What was the diagnosis?
(b) What is the mode of inheritance?
(c) What pathological features were present?
(d) What forms of treatment are available?
(e) What is the immunological defect?

3

Question 1.10

A 28-year-old psychiatrist complains of chest pain on climbing stairs. His 32-year-old brother recently died during a 'fun run'. Despite a normal ECG, cardiac catheterization is performed: left ventricle pressures 170/20 mmHg.

(*a*) What is the most likely diagnosis and one alternative?
(*b*) How could the diagnosis have been substantiated without cardiac catheterization?

Paper 2

Question 2.1

The following data were obtained at cardiac catheterization from a patient aged 22 years known to have had a heart murmur from the age of 3 months:

Chamber	Pressure (mmHg)	Oxygen saturation (%)
Superior vena cava	–	69
Inferior vena cava	–	66
Right atrium	6	67
Right ventricle	120/0	66
Pulmonary artery	150/50	67
Pulmonary artery wedge	8 (mean)	–
Left ventricle	120/0	85
Aorta	120/60	85

What was the diagnosis?

Question 2.2

(a) What is the most common cause of the following arterial blood gas analysis: Po_2 55 mmHg (7.3 kPa); Pco_2 74 mmHg (9.8 kPa); pH 7.27?

(b) What figures will be found in the steady state of the same condition?

Question 2.3

A middle-aged woman was icteric and pruritic. A high titre of antimitochondrial antibodies was demonstrated in her serum.

(a) What was the probable diagnosis?
(b) What would be the histology of a biopsy of the relevant organ?

5

Question 2.4

A 34-year-old man with a hearing aid is seen in outpatients. The following results are found: 24-hour urine protein 1.3 g; mean corpuscular volume (MCV) 106 fl (μm^3); plasma cortisol 60 minutes after synthetic ACTH: 288 nmol/l (10.4 μg/100 ml).

(a) Explain these results.
(b) What diagnosis was made 18 years ago?

Question 2.5

CSF taken from a 25-year-old man with pain, discomfort and weakness of the legs for 4 days showed the following: pressure normal; cells 0.05×10^9/l (50/mm³); protein 0.5 g/l (50 mg/100 ml); VDRL/TPHA negative; culture sterile.

What was the differential diagnosis?

Question 2.6

A 58-year-old man presents with weight loss. The following results are found. Plasma sodium 132, chloride 88, potassium 3.1 mmol/l (mEq/l); serum calcium 3.0 mmol/l (12.1 mg/100 ml).

What is the most likely explanation?

Question 2.7

A woman aged 39 years suffered a hypoplastic anaemia for 3 years which then recovered. Six months later at follow-up the following results were found: Hb 9.5 g/dl (g/100 ml); bilirubin 70 μmol/l (4.1 mg/100 ml); urine contained urobilinogen and haemosiderin; reticulocyte count 12%; red blood cell fragility increased; red blood cell cholinesterase decreased; white blood cell count 2.9×10^9/l (2900/mm³); platelets 100×10^9/l (100 000/mm³).

(a) What was the diagnosis?
(b) What additional investigations are indicated?
(c) What tests will prove the diagnosis?

Question 2.8

A man aged 51 years developed weakness of his legs. Investigations: serum cortisol at 09.00 hours was 1150 nmol/l (41.5 µg/100 ml) and at 24.00 hours 1090 nmol/l (39.5 µg/100 ml). After 48 hours of dexamethasone 8 mg per day the serum cortisol was 1024 nmol/l (37.1 µg/100 ml) at 09.00 hours.

(a) What is the differential diagnosis?
(b) Give two reasons for the weakness of his legs.

Question 2.9

A 67-year-old man with seropositive rheumatoid arthritis developed weakness of dorsiflexion of the right foot, the ankle of which was normal.

(a) What is seropositivity in this context?
(b) How is it mediated?
(c) Name one clinical test which would help clarify the weakness of dorsiflexion.

Question 2.10

A 58-year-old woman with a history of rheumatic fever is admitted semi-conscious and vomiting. An ECG shows runs of ventricular tachycardia and supraventricular tachycardia with varying degrees of heart block. Plasma sodium 148 mmol/l, potassium 6.2 mmol/l, urea 18 mmol/l (108 mg/100 ml).

(a) What is the likely diagnosis and what investigation should be requested immediately?
(b) Why is she so hyperkalaemic?
(c) What is the treatment?

Paper 3

Question 3.1 ✓

The following figures were obtained at cardiac catheterization from a child aged 7 years who was asymptomatic:

Chamber	Pressure (mmHg)	Oxygen saturation (%)
Superior vena cava	–	67
Inferior vena cava	–	69
Right atrium	3.5	68
Right ventricle	35/0	79
Pulmonary artery	35/10	80
Left ventricle	100/0	96

(a) What was the diagnosis?
(b) Describe the physical sign expected.

Question 3.2

A child aged 15 months presented with a history of recurrent respiratory infections. Investigations: Hb 11.0 g/dl (g/100 ml); white blood cell count 17.0 × 10⁹/l (17 000/mm³); neutrophils 70%; lymphocytes 27%; monocytes 2%; eosinophils 1%; sweat sodium 45 mmol/l (mEq/l); serum IgA 0.30 g/l (30 mg/100 ml); IgG 9.0 g/l (900 mg/100 ml); IgM 1.5 g/l (150 mg/100 ml).

(a) What abnormalities were present?
(b) What further investigations would be appropriate?
(c) What is the diagnosis?

8

Question 3.3

A woman aged 45 years had been intermittently icteric for 9 months. Vascular spiders were present. Investigations: serum globulin 63 g/l (6.3 g/100 ml); bilirubin 49.6 μmol/l (2.9 mg/100 ml); aspartate transaminase (AST/SGOT) 120 iu/l; alkalinew phosphatase 128 iu/l (18 King–Armstrong units/100 ml); antinuclear factor (ANF) absent; DNA binding 17%; HBsAg absent; smooth muscle antibodies present 1 in 80; mitochondrial antibodies present 1 in 10; liver biopsy showed piecemeal necrosis, prominent septa and infiltration with lymphocytes and plasma cells.

(a) What was the diagnosis?
(b) What treatment is available?

Question 3.4

During investigation of a hypertensive man with a creatinine clearance of 45 ml/min, urine obtained from bilateral ureteric catheters contained the following:

	Catheter A	Catheter B
Urine volume (ml/min)	2.9	0.6
Urine sodium (mmol (mEq)/min)	0.2	0.08
Urea (mmol/min)	0.19	0.35
(mg/min)	1.09	2.1
Para-aminohippurate (mg/ml)	0.7	2.9

What was the diagnosis?

Question 3.5

A 40-year-old man presents with a flaccid paralysis of the left hand and arm. There is a grasp reflex but no sensory deficit.

(a) Which of the vessels labelled A–J in *Figure 3.1* would you examine closely on the arteriogram and what is it called?
(b) What further clinical feature may be present if the lesion is on the opposite side?

9

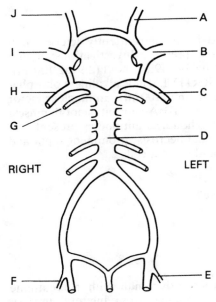

Figure 3.1

Question 3.6

A 64-year-old man has been treated for 2 years for myeloma. He also has a history of peptic ulceration. He is admitted because of malaise and dyspnoea. Hb 45 g/l, white count 6.0×10^9/l, platelets 179×10^9/l, reticulocytes 7%. Pelger cells are seen on the blood film and the marrow shows dyserythropoiesis, plasma cells, stainable iron and ring sideroblasts.

What is the diagnosis?

Question 3.7

A patient aged 55 years with rheumatoid arthritis was found to have the following: Hb 9 g/dl (g/100 ml); MCV 59 fl (μm^3); MCHC 28 g/dl (g/100 ml); reticulocyte count 4%; serum iron 15 μmol/l (84 μg/100 ml); iron binding capacity. 80 μmol/l (444 μg/100 ml)

(*a*) What was the diagnosis?
(*b*) What was the likely cause in this patient?
(*c*) What is the treatment?

Question 3.8

A girl aged 4 years with abnormal facies and on the third percentile for height and tenth percentile for weight was seen for chronic constipation. Investigations: Hb 12.8 g/dl (g/100 ml); serum calcium 1.62 mmol/l (6.48 mg/100 ml); serum phosphate 2.9 mmol/l (8.9 mg/100 ml); plasma creatinine 44 μmol/l (0.5 mg/100 ml).

(a) What was the diagnosis?
(b) Name two further investigations needed.
(c) Name three of the facial features.
(d) Where is the abnormality which underlies this condition?

Question 3.9

A patient with an auto-immune arthropathy developed pericardial and pleural effusions: albumin content 27 g/l (2.7 g/100 ml); glucose concentration 2.1 mmol/l (38 mg/100 ml); C3 10% of normal reference serum; C4 8% of normal reference serum; elongated multinucleate cells were found in the pleural fluid.

(a) What was the diagnosis?
(b) What serum factor would establish the diagnosis?
(c) What type of effusions are these?
(d) What is the differential diagnosis of the pleural effusion?

Question 3.10

A 26-year-old sales representative with a pharmaceutical company complains of diarrhoea. His bowels open four times in the morning before 09.00 hours and then once more in the evening; he does not get up at night to defaecate and there is no blood in the stool. Hb 162 g/l, MCV 89 fl, serum iron 40 μmol/l, total iron binding capacity (TIBC) 60 μmol/l, ferritin 200 μg/l, red cell folate 250 μg/l, serum B$_{12}$ 600 ng/l. The esterified fatty acid 2 hours after a 100 g fat load is 1.2 mmol/l above the fasting concentration.

(a) What is the diagnosis?
(b) What is the treatment?

Paper 4

Question 4.1 ✓

A child aged 10 years was investigated by cardiac catheterization because of a heart murmur. The following data were obtained:

Chamber	Pressure (mmHg)	Oxygen saturation (%)
Superior vena cava	–	63
Inferior vena cava	–	64
Right atrium	2	86
Right ventricle	58/0	90
Pulmonary artery	17/7	89
Femoral artery	101/64	94

What was the diagnosis?

Question 4.2 ✓

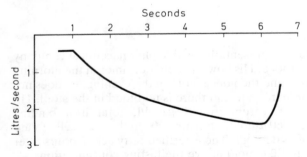

Figure 4.1

The above curve (*Figure 4.1*) was obtained from a man aged 54 years.

12

(*a*) With which group of diseases is the spirogram compatible?
(*b*) Explain the abnormalities.
(*c*) Is the trace compatible with normal arterial pH and blood gases?

Question 4.3

After 3 months of lassitude and amenorrhoea a woman aged 23 years was found to have the following laboratory features: Hb 13.4 g/dl (g/100 ml); white blood cell count $2.9 \times 10^9/l$ (2900/mm³) with a normal differential; plasma bilirubin 100 μmol/l (5.9 mg/100 ml); alanine transaminase (ALT/SGPT) 159 iu/l; aspartate transaminase (AST/SGOT) 390 iu/l; serum albumin 38 g/l (3.8 g/100 ml).

(*a*) What was the diagnosis from the above data?

Further investigations showed: HBsAg absent; serum gamma globulin 60 g/l (6.0 g/100 ml); antinuclear antibody titre 1 in 1024; smooth muscle antibodies present 1 in 264; a high titre of rubella and measles antibodies.

(*b*) What was the diagnosis?
(*c*) What is the prognosis?

Question 4.4

A 59-year-old man was referred to renal outpatients because of proteinuria: 24 h urine 12–15 g protein; protein selectivity 0.7; 24 h glucose excretion 9–11 g.
What was the probable diagnosis?

Question 4.5

A 50-year-old man presents with a dense left-sided hemiplegia and homonymous hemianopia.

(*a*) Which of the vessels labelled A–J in *Figure 4.2* would you examine closely on the arteriogram and what is it called?
(*b*) What further clinical feature may be present if the lesion is on the opposite side?
(*c*) What clinical feature is most important prognostically?

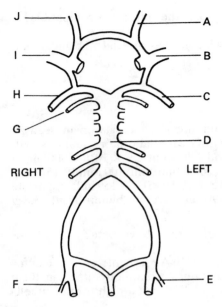

Figure 4.2

Question 4.6

A man aged 75 years who lived alone in a single room complained of increasing back and pelvic discomfort for 18 months. Investigations: creatinine clearance 68 ml/min; serum calcium 2.0 mmol/l (8 mg/100 ml); serum inorganic phosphate 0.6 mmol/l (1.9 mg/100 ml); serum urate 0.4 mmol/l (6.7 mg/100 ml); alkaline phosphatase 127 iu/l (19 King–Armstrong units/100 ml); urine calcium 5.0 mmol/24 h (200 mg/24 h).

(*a*) What was the probable diagnosis?
(*b*) What additional investigations were needed?
(*c*) What treatment is necessary?

Question 4.7

An anaemic patient was treated with oral and subsequently intramuscular iron without improvement: Hb 8.9 g/dl (g/100 ml);

MCHC 27 g/dl (g/100 ml); MCV 69 fl (μm^3); the blood film was hypochromic.

(a) What two diagnoses are possible?
(b) What further investigations are needed?

Question 4.8

A woman of 44 years had a plasma thyroxine of 34.7 nmol/l (2.7 μg/100 ml), fasting plasma thyroid-stimulating hormone (TSH) was not detected. Following intravenous thyrotrophin-releasing hormone (TRH) the plasma TSH was 10 times above normal control values.

(a) What was the diagnosis?
(b) What else should be considered in making the diagnosis?

Question 4.9

A man aged 45 years was admitted to hospital with a blood pressure of 230/140 mmHg and a retinopathy. Despite good control of his blood pressure fresh haemorrhages occurred in the fundi.

(a) What is the principal diagnosis?
(b) Suggest three additional diagnoses.
(c) Suggest investigations to aid your diagnosis.

Question 4.10

A nurse aged 21 years had been febrile and unwell for 12 days when the following investigations became available: bilirubin 85.5 μmol/l (5 mg/100 ml); alanine transaminase (ALT/SGPT) 87 iu/l; alkaline phosphatase 106 iu/l (15 King–Armstrong units/100 ml); urine—bile and urobilinogen present; serum IgM 3.1 g/l (310 mg/100 ml); IgA 1.1 g/l (110 mg/100 ml); IgG 2.0 g/l (2000 mg/100 ml); there was a neutropenia and an absolute lymphocytosis; Hb 10.5 g/dl (g/100 ml); reticulocyte count 6%; Coombs' test positive.

(a) What was the diagnosis?
(b) State two serological confirmatory tests.

Paper 5

From a man aged 50 years with increasing fatigue and dyspnoea
the following data were obtained at cardiac catheterization:

Chamber	Pressure (mmHg)
Right atrium	5
Right ventricle	35/9
Pulmonary artery	35/20
Pulmonary artery wedge	18
Left ventricle	210/9
Left ventricular end diastolic	22
Ascending aorta	142/70

(a) What was the diagnosis?
(b) What is the treatment?

Question 5.2 ✓

The curve shown in *Figure 5.1* was obtained from a man 183 cm tall
aged 39 years.

(a) With what group of diseases is this spirogram compatible?
(b) Will the FEV_1/FVC ratio be abnormal?
(c) Explain the ratio.

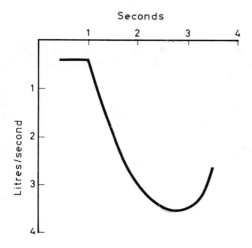

Figure 5.1

Question 5.3

A 43-year-old schizophrenic with jaundice is found to have the
following results: plasma bilirubin 34 μmol/l (2.0 mg/100 ml);
alkaline phosphatase 138 iu/l (19 King–Armstrong units/100 ml);
aspartate transaminase (AST/SGOT) 130 iu/l; γ-glutamyl transpeptidase 58 iu/l; serum albumin 40 g/l (4.0 g/100 ml); mitochondrial and smooth muscle antibodies positive 1 in 2.

(a) What type of jaundice is this?
(b) What would a liver biopsy be likely to show?
(c) Suggest causal agents.

Question 5.4

A boy aged 5 years presented with ascites of 4 days duration. The
plasma albumin was 23 g/l (2.3 g/100 ml) and the urine protein
selectivity was 0.01.

(a) What was the diagnosis?
(b) What is the treatment?
(c) What was the chance of remission with or without treatment?

Question 5.5

A 35-year-old woman taking the oral contraceptive pill complains of blindness in the left eye. Examination shows a left homonymous hemianopia with macular sparing.

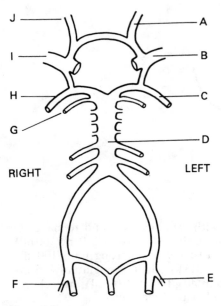

Figure 5.2

Which of the vessels labelled A–J in *Figure 5.2* would you examine closely on the arteriogram and what is it called?

Question 5.6

A man aged 46 years with long-standing back disease and BP 160/50 mmHg had the following investigations: serum calcium 2.0 mmol/l (8 mg/100 ml); serum phosphate 1.9 mmol/l (4.42 mg/ 100 ml); alkaline phosphatase 78 iu/l (11 King–Armstrong units/ 100 ml); serum urate 0.47 mmol/l (7.9 mg/100 ml); blood urea 17.9 mmol/l (118 mg/100 ml)

(*a*) What five further tests are necessary?
(*b*) What was the diagnosis?

18

Question 5.7

A boy aged 4 years was pale and lymph nodes were palpable in his neck. Blood count showed a haemoglobin of 9.0 g/dl (g/100 ml); ESR 40 mm in the first hour (Westergren); white blood cell count 50 × 10⁹/l (50 000/mm³) with a differential count of neutrophils 15%, lymphocytes 12%, lymphoblasts 73%.

(a) What was the diagnosis? Suggest one alternative.
(b) What is the treatment?
(c) What is the prognosis?
(d) List four adverse prognostic features.

Question 5.8

A man aged 29 years presented with visual difficulties, had excessive sweating and an arthropathy. Investigations: creatinine clearance 144 ml/min; urine calcium excretion 9.9 mmol/day (394 mg/day); serum calcium 2.6 mmol/l (10.4 mg/100 ml); serum phosphate 1.7 mmol/l (5.3 mg/100 ml); alkaline phosphatase 106 iu/l (15 King–Armstrong units/100 ml). Treatment was given and all abnormal biochemical measurements became normal in 3 months.

(a) What was the diagnosis?
(b) What additional investigations were essential to make the diagnosis?
(c) How does this condition usually present?

Question 5.9

A man aged 40 years developed persistent heart failure following his first myocardial infarction. There was a long systolic murmur heard over the precordium. Investigations: Hb 11.0 g/dl (g/100 ml); MCHC 30 g/dl (g/100 ml); white blood cell count 13 × 10⁹/l (13 000/mm³); aspartate transaminase (AST/SGOT) 25 iu/l; ECG—sinus rhythm; urine microscopy—red blood cells.

(a) What are the differential diagnoses?
(b) Outline management.

Question 5.10 ✓

A child aged 4 years presented with listlessness. Investigations: Hb 9.5 g/dl (g/100 ml); blood film—much morphological variation between erythrocytes including cigar-shaped cells and target cells; red blood cell osmotic fragility was decreased; haemoglobin electrophoresis abnormal; sodium metabisulphite test positive; reticulocyte count 7–12%; white blood cell count 15 – 10^9/l (15 000/mm³) with a normal differential.

What was the diagnosis?

Paper 6

Question 6.1

The following intra-arterial pressures were recorded from a child aged 2 years, with abnormal facies and a serum calcium of 3.27 mmol/l (13.1 mg/100 ml):

Chamber	Pressure (mmHg)
Left ventricle	140/0
Ascending aorta	140/70
Descending aorta	85/70

What is the differential diagnosis?

Question 6.2

A man aged 42 years had the following results from lung function tests: FEV_1 2.8 litres; FVC 3.1 litres.

(a) What type of lung disease is this?
(b) With what disease is this associated?
(c) Suggest a probable HLA antigen that this man might have.

Question 6.3

An ill-kempt man aged 45 years of no fixed abode was brought to a casualty department by the police. He was semiconscious.

Investigations: plasma sodium 130 mmol/l, potassium 2.9 mmol/l, chloride 71 mmol/l, bicarbonate 40 mmol/l, blood urea 2.3 mmol/l (14 mg/100 ml).

(*a*) What was the diagnosis?
(*b*) Explain the biochemical findings.

Question 6.4 ✓

A 48-year-old Asian woman has the following results: serum calcium 2.0 mmol/l (8 mg/100 ml); alkaline phosphatase 270 iu/l (38 King–Armstrong units/100 ml); 25-OHD$_3$ normal, 1,25-(OH)$_2$D$_3$ and 24,25-(OH)$_2$D$_3$ 20–30% of standard reference sera; intact parathyroid hormone 1200 pg/ml

(*a*) What was the bone disease?
(*b*) What is the explanation?
(*c*) Suggest what the serum inorganic phosphate and urate would be if measured at the same time.

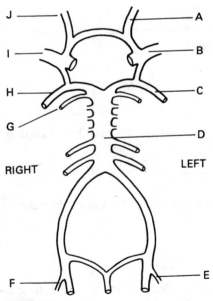

Figure 6.1

22

Question 6.5

A 60-year-old man presents with a collapse. He is deeply unconscious with small fixed pupils. All the limbs are flaccid with bilateral extension plantars.

In which of the labelled vessels in *Figure 6.1* is the lesion likely to be and what is it called?

Question 6.6

A 50-year-old man was admitted because of grossly swollen legs. Investigations: blood volume 68 ml/kg body weight; plasma renin 400 ng ml^{-1}h^{-1}; plasma aldosterone 457 pmol/ml.

Name three illnesses compatible with the above data.

Question 6.7

A man aged 64 years had the following blood count: Hb 10 g/dl (g/100 ml); MCV 110 fl (μm^3); reticulocyte count 1%; target cells were seen on a blood film. Bone marrow was normoblastic and serum vitamin B$_{12}$ was 900 ng/l (pg/ml).

(a) What type of anaemia is this?
(b) What organ needs investigation? List five necessary investigations.

Question 6.8

A man aged 50 years presented with a red face and right heart failure. Symptomatic improvement followed treatment with oral phenoxybenzamine 10 mg three times daily.

(a) What was the diagnosis?
(b) What urinary assay confirms the diagnosis?
(c) Name four other features of this condition.
(d) What other drugs may be of value?

Question 6.9

Following a myocardial infarction a man aged 50 years developed severe angina. Blood pressure 140/90 mmHg. Electrocardiograms showed persistent ST segment elevation in leads V3–V5. The heart was enlarged radiologically with a bulge on the left lateral border.

(*a*) What was the diagnosis?
(*b*) What investigation is required?
(*c*) What are the indications for surgery?

Question 6.10

A girl aged 14 months suffered a cold and mild diarrhoea and vomiting for 20 hours with a little blood in the stools. On admission she was not dehydrated and there were a few petechiae. Investigations: blood urea 10 mmol/l (60 mg/100 ml); plasma sodium 148, potassium 4.5, bicarbonate 18 mmol (mEq/l); Hb 10.2 g/dl (g/100 ml); platelet count $100 - 10^9$/l (100 000/mm^3).

(*a*) Comment on the above figures.
(*b*) What was the diagnosis?
(*c*) What further tests confirm it?
(*d*) Predict the clinical course.

Paper 7

Question 7.1

The following data were obtained from a child aged 4 years with a 47XY karyotype:

Chamber	Pressure (mmHg)	Oxygen saturation (%)
Superior vena cava	–	66
Inferior vena cava	–	70
Right atrium	10	82
Right ventricle	50/0	83
Pulmonary artery	50/25	81
Left atrium	10	95
Left ventricle	95/0	96

(a) What is the cardiac diagnosis?
(b) What is wrong with the child?

Question 7.2

A baby of 35 weeks gestation, birth weight 1.9 kg had a cyanotic attack when 6 hours old. Respiratory rate was 70/min; pulse 140/min; Po_2 75 mmHg (10.0 kPa); Pco_2 50 mmHg (6.6 kPa); pH 7.15; bicarbonate 15 mmol/l (mEq/l).

(a) What was the biochemical disturbance?
(b) What was the differential diagnosis?
(c) What other investigations are essential?

Question 7.3

A life-long teetotal man aged 55 years developed discomfort over his liver 2 days after a myocardial infarction. Investigations: serum albumin 40 g/l (4.0 g/100 ml); alanine transaminase (ALT/SGPT) 43 iu/l, aspartate transaminase (AST/SGOT) 51 iu/l; alkaline phosphatase 120 iu/l (17 King–Armstrong units/100 ml); serum bilirubin 34 μmol/l (2 mg/100 ml); prothrombin time 15 seconds with a control of 13 seconds.

(a) What was the diagnosis?
(b) What treatment was appropriate?

Question 7.4

A Caucasian aged 13 years developed haematuria. Investigations: urine microscopy—granular and red cell casts, sterile on culture; glomerular filtration rate (GFR) 118 ml/min (corrected for surface area); protein excretion 0.2 g/day; serum IgA 158% of normal reference sera; antistreptolysin titre (ASOT) 150 Todd units.

(a) Suggest two possible diagnoses.
(b) What additional features of history were needed?

Question 7.5

A 45-year-old man presents with acute vertigo and dysphagia with regurgitation. He is ataxic and has a small right pupil and right-sided ptosis. There is reduced pinprick sensation on the right side of the face and left side of the trunk and left arm and leg.

(a) Which of the vessels labelled A–J in *Figure 7.1* would you examine closely on the arteriogram and what is it called?
(b) What is this syndrome called?

Question 7.6

A 56-year-old man attends the Casualty Department because of chest pain. He has the following results of investigations: serum osmolarity 290 mmol/l; plasma sodium 150, chloride 106 mmol/l (mEq/l); serum calcium 2.6 mmol/l (10.4 mg/100 ml); serum

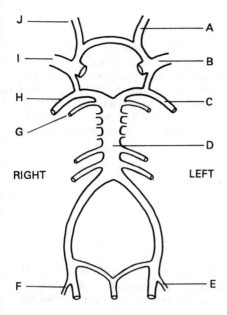

J ——— ——— A

I ——— ——— B

H ——— ——— C

G ——

——— D

RIGHT   LEFT

F ——— ——— E

Figure 7.1

phosphate 1.5 mmol/l (4.6 mg/100 ml); serum albumin 44 g/l (4.4 g/100 ml); blood urea 7.2 mmol/l (47 mg/100 ml); blood glucose 5.2 mmol/l (94 mg/100 ml); plasma potassium 4.0 mmol/l (mEq/l).

(*a*) What is the calculated osmolarity?
(*b*) Explain why the calculated and measured values may differ.

Question 7.7

In a woman aged 68 years with pernicious (Addisonian) anaemia receiving monthly injections of vitamin B_{12} for 11 years, a routine blood count showed: Hb 9 g/dl (g/100 ml); MCHC 26 g/dl (g/100 ml); MCV 67 fl (μm^3); reticulocyte count 0.6%. The blood film showed microcytes.

What was the probable diagnosis?

Question 7.8

A woman aged 45 years presented with weight loss, constipation and vomiting. Investigations: calcium 3.05 mmol/l (12.2 mg/100 ml); plasma phosphate 1.6 mmol/l; alkaline phosphatase 135 iu/l (19 King–Armstrong units/100 ml); random TSH 0.7 mU/l (normal range less than 1.0–3.5 mU/l); a Mantoux test negative; white blood cell count 11.7 − 10^9/l (11 700/mm³), 80% neutrophils, 19% lymphocytes, 1% monocytes. Fasting blood glucose 4.5 mmol/l (81 mg/100 ml).

(a) What was the diagnosis?
(b) Explain the results.

Question 7.9

With what conditions are the following data compatible: pulse 110 beats/min; PR interval 0.22 seconds; erythrocyte sedimentation rate (ESR) 30 mm in the first hour (Westergren); antistreptolysin titre (ASOT) 750 Todd units?

Question 7.10

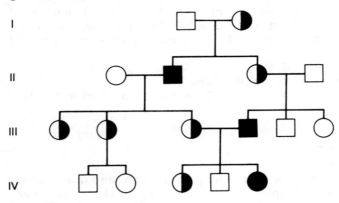

Figure 7.2

(a) What type of inheritance is shown in Figure 7.2?
(b) What unusual event has occurred?
(c) Name three diseases with this inheritance.

Paper 8

Question 8.1

The following data were obtained during cardiac catheterization of a child aged 18 months with a history of cyanotic attacks:

Chamber	Pressure (mmHg)	Oxygen saturation (%)
Superior vena cava	–	67
Inferior vena cava	–	71
Right atrium	4	69
Right ventricle	105/6	70
Pulmonary artery	15/7	69
Left atrium	10	95
Left ventricle	105/0	84
Aorta	105/60	80

(a) What was the diagnosis?

(b) What would a postero-anterior (PA) chest X-ray show?

Question 8.2

Three days after a hip replacement a 60-year-old man with a history of chronic obstructive airways disease is short of breath. Arterial blood gases show: Po_2 80 mmHg (10.6 kPa); Pco_2 37 mmHg (4.9 kPa); pH 7.4. After 40% inspired oxygen for 2 hours the Po_2 was 84 mmHg (11.2 kPa).

(a) What was the differential diagnosis?

(b) What is the explanation?

(c) What test should be performed?

Question 8.3

A man aged 62 years had emergency abdominal surgery for colonic obstruction. Three hours postoperatively he was disproportionately ill. Investigations: Hb 15.9 g/dl (g/100 ml); white blood cell count $17 \times 10^9/l$ (17000/mm^3); platelet count $79 \times 10^9/l$ (79 000/mm^3); plasma fibrinogen 0.05 g/l (50 mg/100 ml); fibrin degeneration products present 1 in 512; blood urea 9.7 mmol/l (64 mg/100 ml).

(a) What was the diagnosis and underlying cause?
(b) Give three other common causes of this problem.
(c) What are two possible complications?

Question 8.4

The following measurements were made in a girl aged 19 years with dependent pitting oedema: urine protein excretion 11.5 g/12 h; urine sodium 8 mmol (mEq) per litre per 12 h; urine calcium 0.3 mmol/24 h; plasma sodium 139 mmol/l (mEq/l); plasma potassium 4.2 mmol/l (mEq/l); serum albumin 23 g/l (2.3 g/100 ml); serum cholesterol 22 mmol/l (851 mg/100 ml); urine microscopy—granular casts and epithelial cells; culture of urine—sterile.

(a) With what condition are these findings compatible?
(b) What will be the urinary aldosterone excretion?

Question 8.5

A boy aged 14 years with a history of a Coombs' negative haemolytic anaemia developed a mixture of parkinsonism and cerebellar ataxia. Investigations showed a generalized amino aciduria; glycosuria; serum urate 100 µmol/l (1.7 mg/100 ml); serum copper 14.4 µmol/l (90 µg/100 ml); urine copper 7130 µmol/24 h (2300 µg/24 h).

(a) What was the diagnosis?
(b) What additional serum measurement was necessary?
(c) What additional physical sign would be expected to be found?

Question 8.6

A 47-year-old man has a serum creatinine 135 μmol/l (1.5 mg/100 ml); AST (SGOT) and ALT (SGPT) normal; total serum protein 60 g/l (6.0 g/100 ml); serum albumin 30 g/l (3.0 g/100 ml); serum urate 0.55 mmol/l (9.2 mg/100 ml); serum calcium 2.7 mmol/l (10.8 mg/100 ml); serum phosphate 1.1 mmol/l (3.4 mg/100 ml); serum cholesterol 8.4 mmol/l (325 mg/100 ml); serum triglyceride 1.95 mmol/l (173 mg/100 ml).

What is the underlying diagnosis and why?

Question 8.7

A woman aged 29 years consulted her general practitioner because of chronic fatigue. The Hb was 8.7 g/dl (g/100 ml); MCHC 26 g/dl (g/100 ml); MCV 63 fl (μm³); reticulocyte count 0.3%; the blood film showed microcytes and hypochromasia. Serum iron 5 μmol/l (28 μg/100 ml) and iron binding capacity 98 μmol/l (498 μg/100 ml).

(a) What was the diagnosis?
(b) Name three common causes in this age group.

Question 8.8

A patient aged 40 years with proven total anterior pituitary failure was treated with thyroxine and cortisol. After an initial improvement he developed nocturia. At 08.00 hours one morning he weighed 73.2 kg, the urine osmolarity was 330 mmol/l and plasma osmolarity 293 mmol/l. Fluid was withheld for 8 hours, when the measurements were repeated: weight was then 69.7 kg, urine osmolarity 239 mmol/l and plasma osmolarity 301 mmol/l

(a) What do these figures demonstrate?
(b) Why did nocturia develop in this man?

Question 8.9

An ECG of a 49-year-old Gibraltarian showed right axis deviation +120° and progressive loss of QRS voltage in the chest leads.

(a) What was the diagnosis?
(b) Name a confirmatory sign.
(c) What other conditions may be found?

Question 8.10

A man aged 71 years was admitted because of deteriorating consciousness. He was found to have hepatosplenomegaly, lymphadenopathy and a retinopathy. Investigations: Hb 9.2 g/dl (g/100 ml); MCHC 30 g/dl (g/100 ml); MCV 79 fl (μm^3); MCH 31 pg ($\mu\mu$g); white cell count 4.1 × 10^9/l (4100/mm^3), differential count normal; ESR 67 mm in the first hour; prothrombin time 17 seconds, control 12 seconds; partial thromboplastin time 44 seconds, control 35 seconds; platelets 125 × 10^9/l (125 000/mm^3); cryoglobulins present; blood viscosity 2.5 × greater than control serum. There was no Bence-Jones proteinuria.

(a) What was the probable diagnosis?
(b) How may this be confirmed?
(c) What retinopathy would one expect to see?
(d) What is the treatment?

Paper 9

Question 9.1

The following pressures were obtained at cardiac catheterization from a woman aged 35 years who had a heart murmur:

Chamber	Pressure (mmHg)
Right atrium	6
Right ventricle	65/0
Pulmonary artery	65/30
Pulmonary artery wedge	18 (mean)
Left ventricle	120/0 to 120/7

(*a*) What was the diagnosis?
(*b*) What may a PA chest X-ray show?

Question 9.2

A man of 61 years who had been previously fit developed wheezing and a productive cough. Chest X-ray—normal; peak flow rate 220 l/min; FEV_1/FVC ratio 42%; following isoprenaline inhalation FEV_1/FVC ratio 54%; sputum contained normal commensal bacteria and eosinophils.

What was the diagnosis?

Question 9.3

A man aged 58 years presented with progressive anorexia and pitting oedema. Investigations: urine normal; alkaline phosphatase 85 iu/l (12 King–Armstrong units/100 ml); alanine transaminase (ALT/SGPT) 20 iu/l; 5-nucleotidase 13 iu/l; total bilirubin 13 μmol/l (0.7 mg/100 ml); serum albumin 27 g/100 ml; clotting studies normal.

What is the probable explanation of these features?

Question 9.4

A 28-year-old woman with a history of renal calculi presents with shortness of breath and generalized weakness. Her electrolytes were: plasma sodium 140 mmol/l (mEq/l); chloride 112 mmol/l (mEq/l); bicarbonate 15 mmol/l (mEq/l); potassium 2.5 mmol/l (mEq/l).

(a) What metabolic abnormalities are present?
(b) What is the differential diagnosis?

Question 9.5

A man aged 67 years developed tender and painful muscles. Investigations: ESR 41 mm in the first hour (Westergren); ANF positive 1:10; sheep cell agglutination test (SCAT) positive 1:4; serum bilirubin 15 μmol/l (0.9 mg/100 ml); serum alanine transaminase (ALT/SGPT) 52 iu/l; LDH 420 iu/l; alkaline phosphatase 85 iu/l (12 King–Armstrong units/100 ml); serum creatine phosphokinase 149 iu/l; total acid phosphatase 9.5 iu/l (5.3 King–Armstrong units/100 ml).

(a) What was the diagnosis?
(b) What two investigations are indicated and what would they demonstrate?

Question 9.6 ✓

A 75-year-old man is seen in the Casualty Department complaining of abdominal pain. He has the following results: blood urea 15.2 mmol/l (91 mg/100 ml) and creatinine 133 μmol/l (1.5 mg/100 ml).

Suggest five explanations for the discrepancy.

Question 9.7 ✓

A boy aged 3 years presented with persistent epistaxis. Hb 12.0 g/dl (g/100 ml); white blood cell count 6.7 × 10^9/l (6700/mm³); platelet count 190 × 10^9/l (190 000/mm³); bleeding and coagulation times normal; prothrombin time 13 seconds with control 12 seconds; PTT (plasma partial thromboplastin time) 70 seconds, control 34 seconds; PTT with 50% normal plasma 43 seconds.

What was the diagnosis?

Question 9.8 ✓

A woman aged 40 years, height 1.75 m, was investigated because of loss of libido and hair together with cold intolerance: serum thyroxine 23 nmol/l (1.8 μg/100 ml); serum TSH 0.2 μg/ml; serum cortisol at 09.00 hours 135 nmol/l (4.9 μg/100 ml); fasting blood glucose 3.4 mmol/l (61 mg/100 ml); plasma ACTH 5 pg/ml; plasma growth hormone fasting 0.8 ng/ml; plasma growth hormone after 1 hour's deep sleep 0.5 ng/ml.

(*a*) What was the diagnosis?
(*b*) List six other features of this condition.

Question 9.9 ✓

Following an episode of loin pain, a 20-year-old man has the DTPA (diethyltriamine pentoacetic acid) renogram shown (*Figure 9.1*).

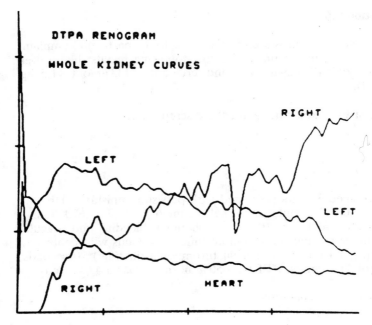

Figure 9.1

(*a*) What does the renogram demonstrate?
(*b*) What treatment is required immediately?
(*c*) After initial treatment what further investigations are needed?

Question 9.10 ✓

A woman aged 33 years with Raynaud's phenomenon of 5 years' duration reported matutinal finger stiffness and dysphagia. Investigations: ESR 71 mm in the first hour (Westergren); Hb 11.9 g/dl (g/100 ml); reticulocyte count 1.3%; ANF positive 1 in 50; cryoglobulins not detected; rheumatoid factor positive 1 in 2; DNA binding 18%. Anticentromere antibodies not detected.

What was the diagnosis?

Paper 10

Question 10.1

The following data were obtained at cardiac catheterization of a child aged 3 years:

Chamber	Pressure (mmHg)	Oxygen saturation (%)
Superior vena cava	10	45
Right atrium	10	44
Right ventricle	95/15	45
Pulmonary artery	20/10	43
Pulmonary artery wedge	15 (mean)	–
Left atrium	–	95

(a) What was the diagnosis?
(b) What feature would one expect to see on a standard chest X-ray?

Question 10.2

The following arterial blood gases were obtained from a 23-year-old man complaining of shortness of breath on exertion: Po_2 102 mmHg (13.6 kPa); arterial oxygen saturation 95%; Pco_2 31 mmHg (4.1 kPa); pH 7.42. After exercise: Po_2 77 mmHg (10.3 kPa); arterial oxygen saturation 85%; Pco_2 29 mmHg (3.8 kPa); pH 7.53.

(a) What was the diagnosis?
(b) How do you explain the changes after exercise?
(c) What confirmatory investigations would be appropriate?

Question 10.3 ✓

A man aged 40 years with coeliac disease controlled with diet developed frequent bowel actions. Faecal fat excretion was more than 20 mmol/day (more than 7 g/day).

(*a*) What were the two most likely diagnoses?
(*b*) How may these diagnoses be made?

Question 10.4 ✓

A 45-year-old man's blood tests reveal: blood urea 14.5 mmol/l (96 mg/100 ml); serum creatinine 495 μmol/l (5.6 mg/100 ml).

(*a*) List four possible explanations of these results.
(*b*) Explain why.

Question 10.5 ✓

Intracranial calcification was seen on the X-ray of a child aged 4 years. The occipital frontal circumference was 48 cm.

List possible causes.

Question 10.6 ✓

A previously healthy man aged 49 years presented with heart failure. Investigations: Hb 14.6 g/dl (g/100 ml); PCV 51%; white blood cell count 10 × 10⁹/l (10 000/mm³), 82% of which were neutrophils; fasting blood glucose 11 mmol/l (198 mg/100 ml); serum albumin 39 g/l (3.9 g/100 ml); serum alanine transaminase (ALT/SGPT), 132 iu/l; serum iron 62.5 μmol/l (350 μg/100 ml); iron binding capacity (TIBC) 70 μmol/l (392 μg/100 ml).

(*a*) What was the diagnosis?
(*b*) List four further clinical features of this condition.

Question 10.7

Three days after a haematemesis in a shipping director aged 32 years the following blood results were reported: Hb 9.5 g/dl (g/100 ml); PCV 32%; MCHC 30 g/dl (g/100 ml); blood film—microcytes, anisocytosis and macrocytosis.

How are these results explained?

Question 10.8

A man aged 41 years with known acromegaly was investigated: serum thyroxine 41 nmol/l (3.2 µg/100 ml); T3 uptake 130%; plasma testosterone 3 nmol/l (0.05 µg/100 ml); serum cortisol at 09.00 hours 40–105 nmol/l (1.4–3.8 µg/100 ml). Fifteen units of soluble insulin and 200 µg TRH were given intravenously. The following results were obtained from blood taken 30 minutes after the intravenous injections: blood glucose 1.9 mmol/l (34 mg/100 ml); growth hormone 0.9 mU/l; plasma cortisol 205 nmol/l (7.4 ng/ml); TSH 5 mU/l.

What were the diagnoses?

Question 10.9

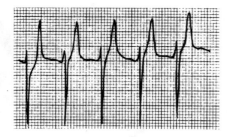

Figure 10.1

(*a*) Comment on the trace (*Figure 10.1*) recorded from a left chest lead.
(*b*) Give two possible diagnoses.

Question 10.10 ✓

Sera from patients A, B and C each agglutinated sheep red blood cells. Separately the sera were then briefly incubated with guinea-pig kidney and beef erythrocytes. Agglutination (+) was then found as shown below:

	Guinea-pig kidney	Beef red blood cells
A	–	+
B	–	–
C	+	–

What were the diagnoses of patients A, B and C?

Paper 11

Question 11.1

Seven years after a heart operation a man developed increasing fatigue, dyspnoea of exertion and paroxysmal nocturnal dyspnoea. Cardiac catheterization data:

Chamber	Pressure (mmHg)
Right atrium	13
Right ventricle	70/8
Pulmonary artery	72/38
Pulmonary artery wedge	25 (mean)
Left ventricle	155/12
Left ventricular end diastolic	9
Aorta	154/80

What was the diagnosis?

Question 11.2

Figures 11.1(a) and *(b)* are pressure/volume curves (lung compliance) obtained from two patients.

(a) What was the diagnosis of patient (a)?
(b) What was the diagnosis of patient (b)?

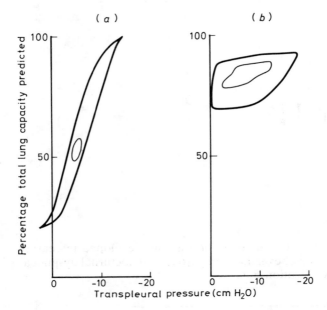

Figure 11.1

Question 11.3

A man aged 54 years presented with dyspnoea of exertion and ascites. The blood pressure was below normal; the heart sounds were soft. Investigations: peak flow rate 480 l/min; Hb and electrolytes normal; blood urea 8 mmol/l (50 mg/100 ml); serum albumin 40 g/l (4.0 g/100 ml); alanine transaminase (ALT/SGPT) 45 iu/l; aspartate transaminase (AST/SGOT) 34 iu/l; serum bilirubin 16 μmol/l (1 mg/100 ml).

What was the cause of the ascites?

Question 11.4

The following results were obtained from a 40-year-old man seen in the Emergency Department because of malaise: Hb 11.9 g/dl (g/100 ml); blood urea 27.5 mmol/l (182 mg/100 ml); plasma creatinine 985 µmol/l (11.1 mg/100 ml); serum urate 0.65 mmol/l (10.9 mg/100 ml); serum calcium 2.01 mmol/l (8.0 mg/100 ml); serum phosphate 2.95 mmol/l (9.1 mg/100 ml); serum magnesium 0.68 mmol/l (1.36 mg/100 ml); serum albumin 39 g/l (3.9 g/100 ml); plasma glucose 6.9 mmol/l (124 mg/100 ml); plasma bilirubin 16 µmol/l (0.9 mg/100 ml); fasting cholesterol 9.1 mmol/l (352 mg/100 ml); fasting triglyceride 4.9 mmol/1 (434 mg/100 ml).

(*a*) Does he have acute or chronic renal failure?
(*b*) Why?

Question 11.5

A woman aged 29 years with a 17-week singleton pregnancy had a serum α-fetoprotein 2.7 times greater than was normal for a comparable woman at that stage of pregnancy.

(*a*) What was the possible diagnosis?
(*b*) What further investigations were necessary?
(*c*) What is the incidence of this condition?

Question 11.6

The following measurements were made in an ill patient: BP 90/50 mmHg; pulse 120 per min; arterial pH 7.22, Po_2 63 mmHg (8.4 kPa); Pco_2 34 mmHg (4.5 kPa); blood lactate 5.9 mmol/l; urine pH 5.2; urine osmolarity 320 mmol/l; blood glucose 8.4 mmol/l (152 mg/100 ml).

(*a*) What was the diagnosis?
(*b*) What underlying conditions could have been present?
(*c*) Can drugs cause this condition?
(*d*) What is the treatment?

Question 11.7

A man aged 60 years who had received ^{32}P for polycythaemia rubra vera 6 years previously, became unwell. Blood examination

showed: Hb 9.8 g/dl (g/100 ml); MCHC 30 g/dl (g/100 ml); MCV
94 fl (μm³); white blood cell count 10 × 10⁹/l (10 000/mm³) with a
differential count of neutrophils 53%, lymphocytes 31%, eosinophils 4%, monocytes 7% and myeloblasts 5%.

(*a*) What was the diagnosis?
(*b*) What would a bone marrow aspirate show?
(*c*) What is the prognosis?

Question 11.8

A woman aged 59 years complained of increasing tiredness for 6
months. Investigations: plasma sodium 130, potassium 6.1,
chloride 96, bicarbonate 23 mmol/l (mEq/l); blood urea 6 mmol/l
(36 mg/100 ml).

(*a*) What was the probable diagnosis?
(*b*) Name one test which will support or refute the diagnosis.

Question 11.9

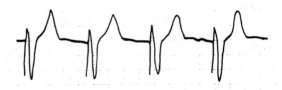

Figure 11.2

What does this ECG strip (*Figure 11.2*) show?

Question 11.10

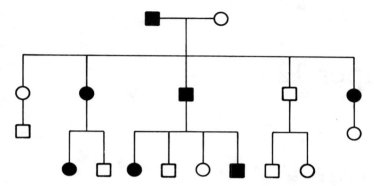

Figure 11.3

(a) What inheritance does this pedigree show?
(b) List five conditions inherited in this manner.

Paper 12

Question 12.1

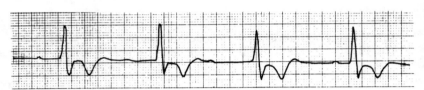

Figure 12.1

The above ECG trace (*Figure 12.1*) was taken from a left chest lead.

(*a*) What was the rhythm?
(*b*) What is the treatment?

Question 12.2

A 28-year-old woman came to the Emergency Department at 06.00 hours because of shortness of breath. Arterial blood gases showed: Po_2 53 mmHg (7.1 kPa); Pco_2 33 mmHg (4.4 kPa); pH 7.28.

With what two diagnoses are these data compatible?

Question 12.3

A woman aged 44 years was admitted to hospital with severe abdominal pain worst to the left. Paralytic ileus was present.

Investigations: blood glucose 8.2 mmol/l (148 mg/100 ml); plasma bilirubin 22 μmol/l (1.3 mg/100 ml); serum calcium 1.85 mmol/l (7.4 mg/100 ml); blood urea 9.5 mmol/l (63 mg/100 ml); methaemalbuminaemia was present.

(a) What was the diagnosis?
(b) What further investigations were needed?
(c) What underlying condition needed to be excluded subsequently?

Question 12.4

A girl aged 18 years with mild oedema had the following findings: blood urea 19.5 mmol/l (128 mg/100 ml); serum albumin 29 g/l (2.9 g/100 ml); urine protein excretion 5–10 g/day.

(a) What was the diagnosis?

Two weeks later her weight had increased by 15 kg. Urine–sterile; protein excretion 25–30 g/day; blood urea 42.8 mmol/l (282 mg/100 ml); serum albumin 21 g/l (2.1 g/100 ml).

(b) What was the probable diagnosis at that stage?
(c) How could it be confirmed?
(d) Outline management.

Question 12.5

The CSF from a 68-year-old retired merchant sailor with a maculopapular reddish rash showed the following: pressure—moderately raised; cells 0.2×10^9/l ($200/mm^3$) predominantly lymphocytes; protein 0.45 g/l (45 mg/100 ml); glucose 3.9 mmol/l (70 mg/100 ml); bacteriological culture sterile.

What is the differential diagnosis?

Question 12.6

Following a herniorrhaphy a man aged 68 years developed a tender swollen knee joint. Investigations: ESR 42 mm in the first hour (Westergren); white blood cell count 13.0×10^9/l

$(13000/mm^3)$ with 79% neutrophils; blood urea 9.9 mmol/l (59 mg/100 ml); serum urate 0.56 mmol/l (9.5 mg/100 ml). Aspiration of the joint fluid showed weak positive birefringence of crystals within a neutrophil.

What was the diagnosis?

Question 12.7

A man of 55 complained of pruritis. The haemoglobin was found to be 18.8 g/dl (g/100 ml); PCV 58%; MCV 80 fl (μm^3); white blood cell count $9.3 \times 10^9/l$ (9300/mm^3) with a normal differential count; the blood film showed a few nucleated red cells. Calcium, phosphate and other electrolytes were normal.

(a) What was the diagnosis?
(b) What four tests are necessary to confirm the diagnosis?
(c) List possible treatments.

Question 12.8

A widow aged 70 years sought advice for tingling and numbness in the fingers. She was also constipated and moderately deaf. All features were of 6 months' duration. Investigations revealed pernicious anaemia and after 6 months of treatment with vitamin B_{12} the anaemia was corrected but her original symptoms were unchanged.

(a) What was the diagnosis?
(b) How is it related to her anaemia?
(c) List 15 further features of this condition.

Question 12.9

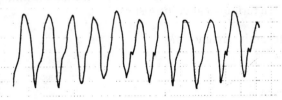

Figure 12.2

(a) What is the probable diagnosis (*Figure 12.2*)?
(b) What feature would be diagnostic?

Question 12.10 ✓

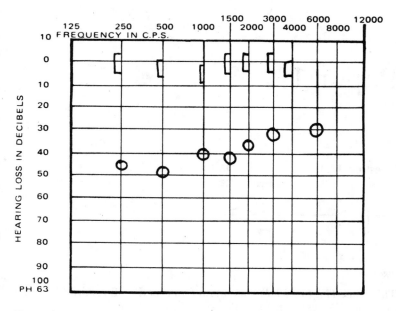

Figure 12.3

A 50-year-old man complains of loss of 20 kg (3 stone) in weight over 4 months. He has fevers and sweats, myalgia and arthralgia. He has noticed a rash, cough, epistaxis and deafness.

(*a*) Of what investigation is this the result?
(*b*) What abnormality does it show?
(*c*) What is the unifying underlying diagnosis?

Paper 13

Question 13.1 ✓

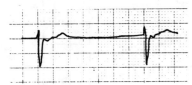

Figure 13.1

This trace (*Figure 13.1*) was taken from lead aVF recorded from a man aged 69 years taking digoxin 0.25 mg daily.

(*a*) What abnormalities were present?
(*b*) What was a probable cause and what other arrhythmias may be seen?

Question 13.2 ✓

A woman aged 19 years had suffered recurrent chest infections for most of her life. Investigations showed: bronchiectasis; FEV_1 0.95 litres; Pco_2 58 mmHg (7.7 kPa).

Name two non-immunological tests which are indicated.

Question 13.3 ✓

A man with severe dyspepsia and diarrhoea had a basal gastric acid secretion of 17 mmol of hydrogen ions in 1 hour. A

50

pentagastrin test did not increase hydrogen ion secretion.

(a) What was the diagnosis?
(b) What other investigations would establish the diagnosis?
(c) What other eponymous syndrome may be present in this patient?

Question 13.4 ✓

The blood urea in a patient with a renal transplant rose from 18.8 mmol/l (113 mg/100 ml) to 35.6 mmol/l (214 mg/100 ml) in 24 hours.

Suggest three causes.

Question 13.5 ✓

A Turkish woman aged 35 years presented with dependent oedema. The past history included multiple attacks of abdominal pain and an arthropathy. Investigations: creatinine clearance 49 ml/min; serum urate 0.38 mmol/l (6.4 mg/100 ml); serum albumin 27 g/l (2.7 g/100 ml); serum cholesterol 14.5 mmol/l (561 mg/100 ml).

(a) What was the immediate diagnosis?
(b) What was the overall diagnosis?
(c) What treatment should be given for (a) and (b)?

Question 13.6 ✓

A 19-year-old Asian immigrant recently arrived in Britain had headaches for 6 weeks and was found unrousable one morning. Investigations: Hb 15.1 g/dl (g/100 ml); white blood cell count 14.9 × 10^9/l (14 900/mm^3) with 77% neutrophils; plasma sodium 150, potassium 4.9, bicarbonate 11 mmol/l (mEq/l); blood urea 13.6 mmol/l (82 mg/100 ml); plasma osmolarity 353 mmol/l; urine osmolarity 770 mmol/l; CSF faintly opalescent and under increased pressure; protein 2.1 g/l (210 mg/100 ml); glucose concentration 17.9 mmol/l (322 mg/100 ml); cell count $0.2 \times 10^9/l$ (200/mm^3) chiefly of neutrophils; Gram stain of CSF—no organisms seen.

(a) What was the blood glucose concentration?
(b) What was the diagnosis?
(c) Comment on the serum and urine osmolarities.

Question 13.7 ✓

A man aged 50 years lost appetite and weight. Blood examinations showed: Hb 10.9 g/dl (g/100 ml); PCV 39%; MCHC 30 g/dl (g/100 ml); white blood cell count $12.8 \times 10^9/l$ (12 800/mm^3), with a differential count of neutrophils 64%, lymphocytes 27%, monocytes 3%, myelocytes 2% and metamyelocytes 4%. Scanning of the blood film showed nucleated red blood cells and platelets were frequent in number.

(a) What is this type of blood picture?
(b) How should it be confirmed?
(c) Name five possible underlying conditions.

Question 13.8 ✓

The following blood glucose concentrations were obtained from venous blood taken from a patient who had been given a 50 g glucose load after an overnight fast:

| | Glucose | |
Time (min)	(mmol/l)	(mg/100 ml)
0	4.5	81
30	11.2	202
60	5.4	97
90	3.3	60
120	4.1	74

(a) What type of curve was this?
(b) Mention three conditions in which it may be found.

Question 13.9

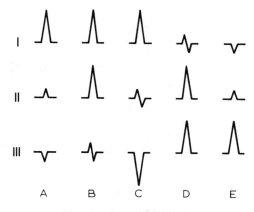

Figure 13.2

Figure 13.2 shows the limb leads I, II, III recorded from five patients.

What are the mean frontal QRS axes of electrocardiograms A, B, C, D and E (*Figure 13.2*)?

Question 13.10

A 17-year-old girl has primary amenorrhoea and short stature. Chest auscultation reveals a murmur and an X-ray is noted to show osteoporosis. Basal LH and FSH are 40 and 30 iU respectively and plasma oestradiol <10 pmol/l.

(*a*) What is the diagnosis?
(*b*) What is the definitive investigation?

Paper 14

Question 14.1

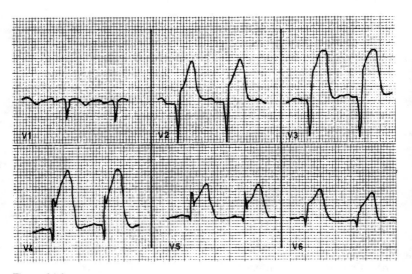

Figure 14.1

This ECG (*Figure 14.1*) was recorded from a woman aged 36 years.

(*a*) What abnormal features are present?
(*b*) What was the diagnosis?
(*c*) Suggest four predisposing factors.

54

Question 14.2 ✓

A farmer aged 34 years complained of worsening episodes of cough and dyspnoea each winter for the past 3 years. Chest X-ray showed fine miliary infiltration; FEV_1 3.0 litres; FVC 3.5 litres; D_{co} (T_{co}) 10 ml min^{-1} per mmHg (predicted 25 ml min^{-1} per mmHg); Po_2 75 mmHg (10 kPa); Pco_2 25 mmHg (3.3 kPa).

(a) What pattern of functional lung abnormality was present?
(b) What was the probable diagnosis?
(c) What is the causal agent?
(d) How is this disease mediated?
(e) What is the treatment?

Question 14.3 ✓

During investigation of a gut disorder a jejunal biopsy was flat when viewed through a dissecting microscope and subtotal villous atrophy was seen histologically.

(a) Name at least two explanations if the patient was a Caucasian child.
(b) Name at least two explanations if the patient was an adult.

Question 14.4 ✓

The following data were obtained from a woman aged 27 years with 'cystitis'; PCV 49%; plasma sodium 140, plasma potassium 7.5, plasma bicarbonate 27, plasma chloride 101 mmol/l (mEq/l); serum calcium 2.55 mmol/l (10.2 mg/100 ml); serum phosphate 0.7 mmol/l (2.2 mg/100 ml).

What was abnormal and what is the probable explanation?

Question 14.5

A woman aged 20 years was admitted because of anxiety depression and a facial rash. There were no focal neurological signs. Investigations: Hb 13.2 g/dl (g/100 ml); white blood cell count 5.0 × 10^9/l (5000/mm³), neutrophils 88%, eosinophils 2%, monocytes 1%, lymphocytes 9%. The EEG showed diffused non-specific findings. Serum C3 29% of normal; ANA diffusely positive, DNA binding 62 U/ml (Amersham).

(a) What was the diagnosis?
(b) What is the treatment?

Question 14.6

In a man aged 40 years fasting plasma stored for 12 hours at 4°C was turbid and had a creamy layer. Cholesterol concentration 12.5 mmol/l (485 mg/100 ml); triglyceride 8.7 mmol/l (770 mg/100 ml); electrophoresis of the lipoproteins showed an abnormal β-lipoprotein.

(a) What type of hyperlipidaemia was this?
(b) What is the metabolic defect?
(c) What clinical manifestations occur?
(d) What treatment is usually recommended?

Question 14.7

A boy aged 10 years developed spontaneous bruising. Many-petechiae were present. Investigations: Hb 14.2 g/dl (g/100 ml); white blood cell count 5.5 × 10^9/l (5500/mm³) with a normal differential; platelets 63 × 10^9/l (63000/mm³); the blood film showed that the platelets were large and misshapen.

(a) What was the diagnosis?
(b) What is the treatment?
(c) If the condition became chronic what additional investigation and treatment would be necessary?

Question 14.8

A man aged 49 years had a haemoptysis and was found to have glycosuria. Plasma potassium 2.9, bicarbonate 33 mmol/l (mEq/l).

(a) What was the diagnosis?
(b) What two further investigations are required?
(c) What is the prognosis?

Question 14.9 ✓

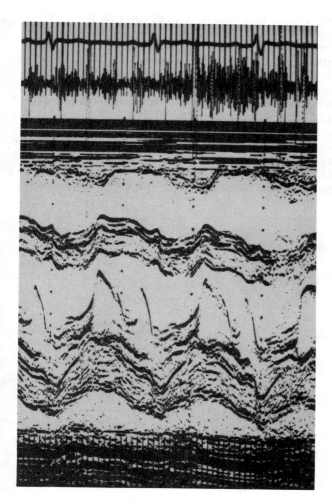

Figure 14.2

Figure 14.2 is an echocardiogram recorded in an adult.

(a) What abnormality is present?
(b) What might the chest X-ray show?

Question 14.10

A patient with a GFR of 5 ml/min developed bone pain. Serum calcium 2.1 mmol/l (8.3 mg/100 ml); phosphate 3.3 mmol/l (10.3 mg/100 ml); alkaline phosphatase 270 iu/l (35 King–Armstrong units/100 ml). He was subsequently treated with alfacalcidol in a dose of 2 μg orally daily. He was seen 6 months later. Investigations: serum calcium 3.55 mmol/l (14.2 mg/100 ml); serum phosphate 2.96 mmol/l (9.2 mg/100 ml); alkaline phosphatase 135 iu/l (19 King–Armstrong units/100 ml).

(a) What was the original diagnosis?
(b) What was the subsequent diagnosis?
(c) Comment upon management.
(d) What complications may result from the above sequence of events?

Paper 15

Question 15.1 ✓

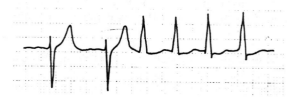

Figure 15.1

What does this rhythm strip (*Figure 15.1*) show?

Question 15.2 ✓

The following results were obtained from a patient who had had a partial gastrectomy 2 days previously: plasma sodium 75, potassium 2.7, bicarbonate 13 mmol/l (mEq/l); total protein 63 g/l (6.3 g/100 ml).

What was the diagnosis?

Question 15.3 ✓

A 39-year-old man awaiting a hip replacement gives a history of recurrent abdominal pain and is found to have a spleen extending

59

10 cm below the right costal margin. Total acid phosphatase is 12 iu/l and prostatic acid phosphatase 1 iu/l.

(a) What is the diagnosis?
(b) What is his likely ethnic origin?
(c) What haematological test is most relevant pre-operatively?

Question 15.4

A 56-year-old divorcée with four children has recently noticed weight loss, tiredness, malaise, nocturia and pruritis. Her BP is 170/100 and she has persistent sterile pyuria. Hb 760 g/l, MCV 73 fl, urea 15 mmol/l (90 mg/100 ml), creatinine 600 μmol/l (6.9 mg/100 ml). A high-dose intravenous urogram shows small kidneys, deformed calyces and a filling defect at the right pelvis on some films.

(a) What is the diagnosis and aetiology and what complication may have occurred?
(b) What two tests should be performed?

Question 15.5

A previously fit 18-year-old man was drowned. Venous blood taken just before death showed: Hb 9.8 g/dl (g/100 ml); PCV 41%; plasma sodium 123, potassium 6.7, chloride 85 mmol/l (mEq/l); serum magnesium 0.82 mmol/l (1.96 mg/100 ml); arterial P_{O_2} 59 mmHg (7.9 kPa); P_{CO_2} 67 mmHg (8.9 kPa); pH 7.26.

(a) Did this patient die of inhalation of fresh or sea water?
(b) What terminal arrhythmia did he have?

Question 15.6

A hypertensive West Indian receiving diazoxide therapy was admitted semicomatose. Investigations: blood glucose 70 mmol/l (1260 mg/100 ml); plasma sodium, potassium and urea 155,

3.2 mmol/l (mEq/l) and 8.4 mmol/l (55 mg/100 ml) respectively. There was no ketonuria.

(*a*) What was the diagnosis?
(*b*) What was the plasma osmolarity?
(*c*) How does treatment differ from that of diabetic ketoacidosis?

Question 15.7

The following results are found in a man aged 59 years: MCV 110 fl (μm^3); Hb 12.5 g/dl (g/100 ml); vitamin B_{12} 750 ng/l (750 pg/ml); serum albumin 33 g/l (3.3 g/100 ml); serum calcium 2.95 mmol/l (11.8 mg/100 ml); serum urate 0.54 mmol/l (9.2 mg/100 ml); plasma creatinine 305 $\mu mol/l$ (3.5 mg/100 ml); λ and $\varkappa$ chains in the urine; IgG concentration 41 g/l (4.1 g/100 ml).

(*a*) What is the diagnosis?
(*b*) Explain all the results given.
(*c*) What is the prognosis?
(*d*) What two drugs are most commonly used in treatment?

Question 15.8

Investigation of a 58-year-old man complaining of arthritis, bloody diarrhoea and weight loss shows: faecal fat excretion 149 mmol (42 g) over a 3-day period; creatinine clearance 40 ml/min; urine protein 1.8 g/24 h; Howell–Jolly bodies on the blood film; 30% prolongation of prothrombin time and partial thromboplastin time but normal thrombin time.

What is the diagnosis?

Question 15.9

At a routine medical examination a 25-year-old man gives a history of abdominal pain. No gallstones are seen on oral cholecystogram, neither is his gallbladder opacified. Urine testing shows bilirubin and urobilinogen. The ratio of coproporphyrin I to coproporphyrin III in the urine is 5:1 (normal 1:3).

(a) What is the diagnosis?
(b) What is the inheritance of this condition?
(c) In the past what further test may have been performed to confirm the diagnosis?

Question 15.10

A 48-year-old woman who had a renal transplant 4 years previously presents with a 2-week history of nausea, vomiting and malaise. Investigations show blood glucose 2.5 mmol/l (45 mg/100 ml); plasma sodium 125 mmol/l; blood urea 3.8 mmol/l (22.8 mg/100 ml); plasma creatinine 150 µmol/l (1.7 mg/100 ml).

What is the differential diagnosis?

Paper 16

Question 16.1

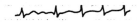

Figure 16.1

(*a*) What is this rhythm (*Figure 16.1*)?
(*b*) List six possible causes.

Question 16.2

An 18-year-old girl is found to have: blood glucose 10.8 mmol/l (196 mg/100 ml); plasma potassium 6.5 mmol/l (mEq/l); blood urea 4.7 mmol/l (28 mg/100 ml); plasma noradrenaline 805 pg/ml; urine metanephrines 17 μmol/24 h (3.1 mg/day); urinary hydroxy-methoxymandelic acid 52 μmol/24 h (10.3 mg/day).

(*a*) With what diagnosis are the above data compatible?
(*b*) How might she have presented?
(*c*) How may the site of the lesion be identified?

Question 16.3

A 21-year-old man has a haematemesis. There is a history of recurrent chest infections and his younger brother died at the age of 10 years. His genotype is PiZZ.

(*a*) Of what substance is he deficient?
(*b*) How deficient is he (what percentage of the normal level)?
(*c*) What is the gene frequency in this condition?
(*d*) What is the treatment of choice and what four other conditions may be treated this way?

Question 16.4 ✓

A 60-year-old insulin-dependent diabetic presents to Casualty with a history of diarrhoea, vomiting and muscle weakness. He has claudication and 2 years ago had an inferior myocardial infarct. Plasma sodium 134 mmol/l; potassium 7.3 mmol/l; bicarbonate 10 mmol/l; chloride 120 mmol/l; urea 20 mmol/l (120 mg/100 ml); serum creatinine 550 µmol/l (5.1 mg/100 ml).

(*a*) What is the diagnosis?
(*b*) What is the pathophysiology?
(*c*) What is the treatment?

Question 16.5 ✓

A man with Q waves in leads II, III and aVF was found to have a fasting serum cholesterol of 11.8 mmol/l (457 mg/100 ml), the triglyceride concentration being 1.53 mmol/l (136 mg/100 ml) together with an excess of low density lipoproteins (LDL).

(*a*) What is the name of this lipid disorder?
(*b*) Would xanthomata be present?
(*c*) What occurs if serum from such a patient is stored for 18 hours at 4°C?

Question 16.6 ✓

Four days after a suicide attempt the following investigations were available: Hb 12.0 g/dl (g/100 ml); white blood cell count 17.5 × 10^9/l (17 500/mm^3) with 89% neutrophils; serum phosphate 2.3 mmol/l (7.1 mg/100 ml); serum calcium 2.5 mmol/l (10 mg/ 100 ml); blood urea 17.2 mmol/l (103 mg/100 ml); arterial pH 7.23;

plasma bilirubin 123 μmol/l (7.2 mg/100 ml); alanine transaminase (SGPT) 392 iu/l; prothrombin time 21 seconds, control 14 seconds; alkaline phosphatase 78 iu/l (11 King–Armstrong units/100 ml).

Name two compounds that this patient could have taken.

Question 16.7

An English child aged 3 years who had been taken to various Mediterranean and African resorts twice annually presented with epistaxis, weight loss, lymphadenopathy, swollen abdomen and irritability. Investigations: Hb 9.9 g/dl (g/100 ml); MCHC 30 g/dl (g/100 ml); MCV 77 fl (μm^3); platelets 99 × 10^9/l (99 000/mm^3); white blood cell count 2.9 × 10^9/l (2900/mm^3), 87% lymphocytes; serum IgG 61.0 g/l (6100 mg/100 ml); Coombs' test positive; bone marrow—normoblastic, no leukaemic changes but clusters of ovoid bodies 2–4 μm in diameter containing two masses of chromatin material were present.

What was the diagnosis?

Question 16.8

A boy aged 7 months had suffered recurrent ear, throat and chest infections: peripheral white blood cell count 3 × 10^9/l; bone marrow aspiration normal; differential B- and T-cell counts normal; measurements of phagocytosis of *Candida albicans* spores normal; estimation of lymphokine function normal; skin testing for dinitrochlorobenzene sensitivity normal.

What is the diagnosis?

Question 16.9

A 34-year-old Chinese primigravida with a singleton pregnancy has a serum α-fetoprotein (measured at 16 weeks gestation) that is six times the upper limit of normal.

(*a*) What is the differential diagnosis?
(*b*) What further investigations are required?

Question 16.10

A 10-year-old boy has a squint and early cataract formation. He is of short stature, has a round face, a short neck and stubby hands. Investigations: serum calcium 2.2 mmol/l; serum phosphate 1.2 mmol/l; serum creatinine 60 μmol/l (0.7 mg/100 ml).

What is the diagnosis?

Paper 17

Question 17.1

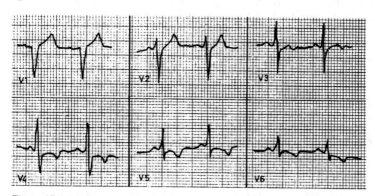

Figure 17.1

What do these chest leads (*Figure 17.1*) show?

Question 17.2

The following venous blood glucose concentrations were found after a 50 g glucose load was given to a woman aged 39 years after she had fasted overnight.

Name two conditions compatible with these figures.

67

Time (min)	Glucose (mmol/l)	(mg/100 ml)
0	4.3	77
30	6.3	113
60	6.9	124
90	4.9	88
120	4.4	79

Question 17.3 ✓

A 48-year-old man of no fixed abode is released from prison in June. He attends the Casualty Department in early August complaining of itchy blisters on his face, bald pate, hands and forearms. Hb 13 g/dl; mean cell volume (MCV) 100 fl; urinary uroporphyrin 120 nmol/day (normal < 49); urinary δ-aminolaevulinic acid (ALA) 30 μmol/day (normal < 40).

(a) What is the diagnosis?
(b) What is the likely precipitating cause?
(c) What is the treatment?

Question 17.4 ✓

Three weeks after receiving a cadaveric renal transplant a 19-year-old man's results are: plasma sodium 140 mmol/l; potassium 6.8 mmol/l; bicarbonate 13 mmol/l; chloride 114 mmol/l; urea 12 mmol/l (72 mg/100 ml); creatinine 175 μmol/l (2 mg/100 ml).

(a) What is the diagnosis?
(b) What is the pathophysiology?
(c) What drug is he likely to be taking?
(d) What is the treatment?

Question 17.5 ✓

These tracings (*Figure 17.2*) were obtained from a 38-year-old woman who complained of tripping over her right foot and numbness of her left index finger.

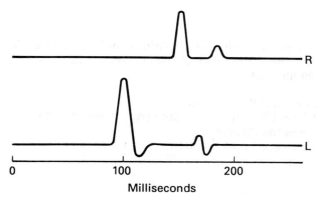

Figure 17.2

(a) What test was performed?
(b) What do the tracings show and what is the diagnosis?

Question 17.6

An infant aged 11 months was admitted as a 'failure to thrive'. He passed large urine volumes and had a normal blood pressure. Investigations: plasma sodium 140, potassium 2.3, bicarbonate 31 mmol/l (mEq/l); blood urea 2.8 mmol/l (18 mg/100 ml); plasma renin activity was very high as was plasma angiotensin II. Urinary aldosterone and prostaglandin levels were supranormal.

(a) What was the diagnosis?
(b) What morphological confirmation could be obtained?
(c) What is the treatment?

Question 17.7

Measurements made from cord blood of a second child of an unbooked mother aged 26 years were: Hb 13.0 g/dl (g/100 ml); bilirubin 65 μmol/l (3.8 mg/100 ml); blood group B, Rhesus positive to anti-D.

(a) What was the probable diagnosis?
(b) What is the differential diagnosis?
(c) What further investigations were necessary?

Question 17.8

During investigation of a rash, a biopsy from an uninvolved area of skin was taken. Immunofluorescence demonstrated the presence of immunoglobulins and C3.

(*a*) Suggest four possible diagnoses.
(*b*) If a small bowel biopsy in the same patient showed blunted villi, what was the diagnosis?
(*c*) What is the treatment of the dermatological problem?

Question 17.9

A 19-year-old girl has primary amenorrhoea and poor breast development. She is 6 ft 1 in (175 cm) tall and has scanty axillary and pubic hair. Plasma LH 11 iU/l; FSH 61 iU/l; prolactin 5.5 µg/l; testosterone 0.8 nmol/l; oestradiol <100 pmol/l (normal 150–870 pmol/l).

(*a*) What is the differential diagnosis from the history?
(*b*) What diagnosis do the results support?

Question 17.10

A 20-year-old man presents with polyuria, erectile failure, reduction in beard growth and shortness of breath. Serum iron 70 µmol/l; total iron binding capacity (TIBC) 72 µmol/l; ferritin 2000 µg/l.

(*a*) What is the diagnosis?
(*b*) Explain the presenting complaints.
(*c*) What treatments are available?

Paper 18

Question 18.1

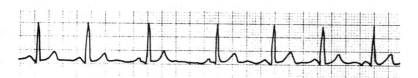

Figure 18.1

(*a*) What is this rhythm (*Figure 18.1*)?
(*b*) State four possible causes.

Question 18.2

At 56 hours post-hysterectomy for a cervical carcinoma an obese woman aged 59 years was noted to have a respiratory rate of 31/min. Investigations: ECG rate 120/min otherwise normal; chest X-ray showed atelectasis at the right base; Hb 9.8 g/dl (g/100 ml); Po_2 54 mmHg (7.2 kPa); Pco_2 24 mmHg (3.2 kPa); bicarbonate 30 mmol/l (mEq/l); pH 7.57.

(*a*) What does the arterial sample show?
(*b*) What was the differential diagnosis?

71

Question 18.3

A man aged 60 years underwent a technically difficult cholecystectomy. Two days postoperatively jaundice developed. On day 7 the following investigations were reported: serum bilirubin 667 µmol/l (39 mg/100 ml); serum alkaline phosphatase 89 iu/l (12.5 King–Armstrong units/100 ml); aspartate transaminase (AST/SGOT) 95 iu/l; alanine transaminase (ALT/SGPT) 102 iu/l; HBsAg negative; prothrombin time 17 seconds, control 13 seconds.

Suggest two possible diagnoses.

Question 18.4

The following measurements were made on a 'random' urine sample from a patient who had recently become oliguric: sodium 92 mmol/l (mEq/l); osmolarity 312 mmol/l; urea 75 mmol/l (450 mg/100 ml); Blood taken at the same time showed: plasma sodium 142 mmol/l (mEq/l); potassium 5.3 mmol/l (mEq/l); bicarbonate 23 mmol/l (mEq/l); blood urea 10.8 mmol/l (65 mg/100 ml); osmolarity 288 mmol/l.

(a) What was the diagnosis?
(b) Would the patient respond with a diuresis to intravenous saline and a 'loop' diuretic?
(c) What further two investigations may be valuable?

Question 18.5

A 50-year-old woman with white hair complains of shortness of breath on exertion and of being unsteady on her feet. She has a central venous pressure of +10 to 15 cmH$_2$O, a cardiac output of 1.4 l/min and a motor conduction time of 20 m/s.

Give four possible diagnoses.

Question 18.6

A 26-year-old nurse is brought to Casualty unconscious. Plasma sodium 145, potassium 5.0, chloride 98, bicarbonate 20 mmol/l (mEq/l).

72

(*a*) What is the anion gap from the above figures?
(*b*) What constitutes the gap?
(*c*) What is the differential diagnosis?

Question 18.7

A patient had an ileal resection for Crohn's disease. One year later the haemoglobin was found to be 9.2 g/dl (g/100 ml); reticulocyte count 1.3%; MCV 118 fl (μm³); MCH 39 pg ($\mu\mu$g); platelets 100 × 10⁹/l (100 000/mm³); white blood cell count 1.5 × 10⁹/l (1500/mm³) with a neutropenia; serum vitamin B_{12} 79 ng/l (pg/ml); serum folate 15 μg/l (ng/ml); antibodies to gastric parietal cells positive 1 in 128; bone marrow aspirate showed megaloblastic changes. A Schilling test showed low urinary excretion of labelled vitamin B_{12} when the vitamin was given alone and with intrinsic factor.

(*a*) What was the diagnosis?
(*b*) How could this be tested easily?

Question 18.8

A healthy insulin-dependent diabetic aged 23 years attended her doctor because of recent evening fainting attacks. Testing of urine at the time of these episodes showed 0.75–1% glycosuria. She had not recently changed her dose of insulin. Blood glucose concentrations at 08.00, 12.00, 16.00 and 20.00 hours the following day were 10.3 (185), 13.2 (237), 6.8 (123) and 4.7 (85) mmol/l (mg/100 ml) respectively.

(*a*) What was the diagnosis?
(*b*) What underlying condition was present?

Question 18.9

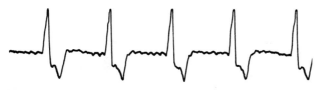

Figure 18.2

73

Figure 18.2 is the trace obtained from lead V4 in a man aged 63 years.

(*a*) What arrhythmia is present?
(*b*) What treatment is required?

Question 18.10 ✓

A woman was admitted after an overdose. She was given an injection, recovered consciousness and discharged herself. Six days later she was readmitted: alanine transaminase (ALT/SGPT) 956 iu/l; bilirubin 123 μmol/l (7.2 mg/100 ml); alkaline phosphatase 159 iu/l (22.4 King–Armstrong units/100 ml); serum creatinine 199 μmol/l (2.6 mg/100 ml).

(*a*) What comprised the overdose?
(*b*) What injection was she given?

Paper 19

Question 19.1

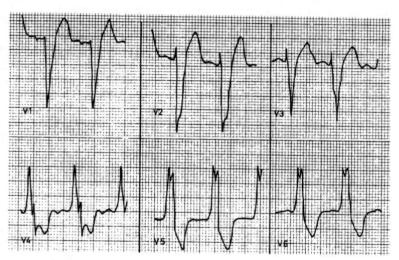

Figure 19.1

(*a*) What abnormalities do these precordial leads show?
(*b*) Suggest three possible causes.

Question 19.2

A homeless single man aged 50 years attended the Accident and Emergency Department complaining of haemoptysis. A chest

75

X-ray showed old multiple rib fractures and extensive mottling of the lungs.

(*a*) What was the diagnosis?
(*b*) What abnormal results may be expected from the laboratory investigations?

Question 19.3

A man aged 61 years was admitted to hospital with a 4-hour history of abdominal pain and vomiting. Investigations: Hb 21.5 g/dl (g/100 ml); PCV 68%; white blood cell count 12 × 10^9/l (12 000/mm³); platelet count 570 × 10^9/l (570 000/mm³); ESR 3 mm in the first hour; serum amylase 150 iu/l; alanine transaminase (ALT/SGPT) 95 iu/l; alkaline phosphatase 163 iu/l (23 King–Armstrong units/100 ml); serum albumin 36 g/l (3.6 g/ 100 ml); serum bilirubin 29 μmol/l (1.7 mg/100 ml); liver isotope scan—generally poor uptake with excess uptake in the caudate lobe.

(*a*) What was the primary diagnosis?
(*b*) What complication had occurred?
(*c*) What other signs would be expected to develop?
(*d*) What further investigation would be necessary?

Question 19.4

A Caucasian man aged 29 years was found to have a blood pressure of 170/115 mmHg. Plasma renin was 37 pg ml plasma^{-1}h^{-1} and plasma aldosterone 1590 pmol/l. He was given a 10 mmol (mEq) sodium diet for 5 days. At the end of this period the plasma renin and plasma aldosterone were unchanged.

(*a*) What was the diagnosis?
(*b*) Name two further investigations.
(*c*) What is the treatment?

Question 19.5

A 30-year-old man complained of difficulty in walking. CSF showed the following: colour xanthochromic; pressure 14 cmH$_2$O;

protein 4.9 g/l (490 mg/100 ml); glucose 4.1 mmol/l (74 mg/100 ml); cells 2 lymphocytes/mm^3; culture was reported as sterile.

(*a*) What was the diagnosis?
(*b*) What was the differential diagnosis?

Question 19.6 ✓

A previously healthy woman aged 24 years was found to have hypertension, oedema of the ankles and abdominal distension. Investigations: reducing substance present in urine; proteinuria 3–4 g/day; creatinine clearance 78 ml/min; serum urate 0.59 mmol/l (9.2 mg/100 ml). Shortly after these findings the patient suffered a convulsion.

What was the most likely diagnosis?

Question 19.7 ✓

A man aged 73 years had the following findings: Hb 8.2 g/dl (g/100 ml); blood film—normochromic and hypochromic cells; reticulocyte count 0.7%. Oral iron was given for 6 weeks without increase in the haemoglobin. Further investigations: faecal occult blood not detected; barium meal and enema normal; serum iron 45 μmol/l (252 μg/100 ml); iron binding capacity 90 μmol/l (500 μg/100 ml); MCHC 30 g/dl (g/100 ml); white blood cell count 4.7 × 10^9/l (4700/mm^3) with a normal differential.

(*a*) What was the probable diagnosis?
(*b*) What would a bone marrow aspiration show?
(*c*) What are the possible causes?

Question 19.8 ✓

An inquisitive medical student sent her own blood for thyroid function tests which were reported as follows: thyroxine (T4) 178 nmol/l (13.8 μg/100 ml); T3 resin uptake 83% (supernatant not counted).

Give two explanations.

Question 19.9

A woman aged 26 years, having had active Still's disease since the age of 10, developed increased ankle oedema. Investigations: ESR 60 mm in the first hour (Westergren); Hb 10.7 g/dl (g/100 ml); MCHC 30 g/dl (g/100 ml); MCH 31 pg (μμg); 24 hour urine protein excretion 13.7 g; creatinine clearance 39 ml/min; plasma albumin 27 g/l (2.7 g/100 ml); urine was found to contain free λ and ϰ chains; serum immunoglobulins within normal range; rheumatoid factor absent; IVP normal gross anatomy of urinary tract.

(a) What was the main functional renal diagnosis?
(b) Suggest two likely causes.
(c) Suggest two further investigations.

Question 19.10

A severe epileptic aged 30 years gradually developed backache. Investigations: blood urea 3.9 mmol/l (25.7 mg/100 ml); serum albumin 40 g/l (4.0 g/100 ml); serum calcium 2.1 mmol/l (8.4 mg/ 100 ml); serum inorganic phosphate 0.9 mmol/l (2.8 mg/100 ml); plasma alkaline phosphatase 177 iu/l (25 King–Armstrong units/100 ml); plasma 25-OHD₃ 43% of standard reference sera.

(a) What was the diagnosis?
(b) Why had it occurred?
(c) What is the pathogenesis?

Paper 20

Questin 20.1

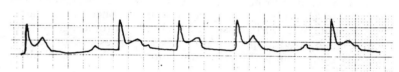

Figure 20.1

(*a*) What arrhythmia is this (*Figure 20.1*)?
(*b*) What other condition is present?

Question 20.2

A woman 23 years of age with arthropathy developed a pleural effusion. Investigations: pleural fluid hazy, containing a few lymphocytes; pH 7.15; glucose 1.3 mmol/l (23 mg/100 ml); protein 48 g/l (4.8 g/100 ml); specific gravity 1.024; circulating immune complexes present; C_3 <0.1 g/l.

(*a*) What is the diagnosis?
(*b*) What would be the concentration of the pleural fluid lactic acid dehydrogenase (LDH)?

Question 20.3

The following investigations were obtained from a woman aged 56 years: serum bilirubin 50 μmol/l (2.9 mg/100 ml); alanine transaminase (ALT/SGPT) 25 iu/l; serum alkaline phosphatase 772 iu/l

(110 King–Armstrong units/100 ml); serum copper 31.2 µmol/l (195 µg/100 ml); serum ceruloplasmin 2 µmol/l (30 mg/100 ml); urine copper 264 µmol/24 hours (85 µg/24 hours); liver copper 985 µg/g dry weight (normal 18–45 µg/g dry weight).

(a) What was the diagnosis?
(b) How might it be confirmed?

Question 20.4 ✓

During the investigation of a proteinuria of 1.3 g/day in a man aged 40 years the following results were obtained: plasma pH 7.35; persistent glycosuria; plasma phosphate 0.5 mmol/l (1.55 mg/ 100 ml); maximum urine acidity after 0.1 g/kg bodyweight load of ammonium chloride 5.9; maximum urinary concentration after dehydration and vasopressin 499 mmol/l; chromatography of urine—generalized amino-aciduria; electrophoresis of urine protein—little albumin and increased quantities of β-microglobulin.

(a) What was the diagnosis?
(b) What type of curve would be obtained if a GTT were performed in this man?

Question 20.5 ✓

A 19-year-old man attending the Casualty Department for removal of sutures complains of poor vision. The visual fields are shown in *Figure 20.2*.

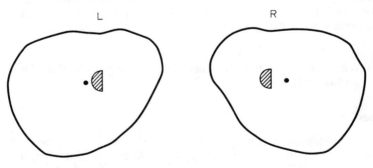

L   R

Figure 20.2

(*a*) What is the name of the defect shown in *Figure 20.2*?
(*b*) What is the anatomical site of the lesion?
(*c*) What causes such lesions?

Question 20.6

A child aged 1 year presented with global retardation and subsequently developed choreo-athetosis and spasticity. He had features of compulsive self-mutilation. By the age of 5 years he had developed an arthropathy and a macrocytic anaemia. Investigations: blood urea 3.7 mmol/l (22 mg/100 ml); serum urate 0.83 mmol/l (13.9 mg/100 ml); serum calcium 2.5 mmol/l (10.1 mg/ 100 ml); serum phosphate 0.71 mmol/l (2.2 mg/100 ml).

(*a*) What was the diagnosis?
(*b*) What is the cause of this condition?

Question 20.7

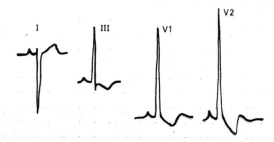

Figure 20.3

The ECG in *Figure 20.3* was obtained from a man aged 53 years with a Hb of 20 g/dl (g/100 ml) and a red blood cell count of $7.1 \times 10^{12}/l$ ($7.1 \times 10^6/mm^3$).

(*a*) What does the ECG show?
(*b*) Name two possible associations between the ECG and the haematological findings.

81

Question 20.8

A man aged 45 years with treated moderate hypertension left for a business trip. About 36 hours after leaving home he attended a casualty department complaining of headache, agitation, sweating and palpitations. The blood pressure was 220/145 mmHg. He was admitted and investigations showed a urinary catecholamine excretion of 15 µmol/24 hours (274 mg/24 hours).

(*a*) What was the differential diagnosis?
(*b*) What hypotensive agent had he left at home?
(*c*) What is the treatment of this condition and with what drug?

Question 20.9

A woman aged 76 years who had morning stiffness with pectoral and pelvic girdle pain for 9 months suddenly developed severe right temporal pain and noted rapid deterioration of vision in the right eye. The ESR was 98 mm in the first hour (Westergren).

(*a*) What was the diagnosis?
(*b*) How may the diagnosis be confirmed?
(*c*) What is the treatment?
(*d*) When should treatment be started?

Question 20.10

A 26-year-old man with a history of loin pain is found to have a low urinary urate concentration and a 24 h urinary calcium excretion of 2.0 mmol.

(*a*) What drug is he taking?
(*b*) What metabolic diseases may be associated with this group of drugs?
(*c*) In what condition is one of these properties of therapeutic value?

Paper 21

Question 21.1

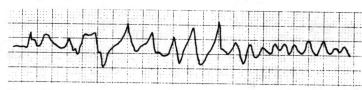

Figure 21.1

(a) What arrhythmias are present (*Figure 21.1*)?
(b) What is the treatment?

Question 21.2

A man with an acute exacerbation of chronic bronchitis was admitted to hospital and received treatment. After 6 hours he was found to have deteriorated. Arterial blood findings were: P_{O_2} 108 mmHg (14.4 kPa); P_{CO_2} 141 mmHg (18.8 kPa); pH 7.21.

(a) What was the diagnosis?
(b) What error in treatment had been made?
(c) What physical signs are likely to be present?
(d) Outline further treatment.

Question 21.3

An asymptomatic executive aged 40 years had a series of biochemical measurements as a routine procedure upon joining a new firm. Among his measurements the serum bilirubin was found to be 30 μmol/l (1.8 mg/100 ml); serum albumin 42 g/l (4.2 g/100 ml); alanine transaminase (ALT/SGPT) 15 iu/l; alkaline phosphatase 85.5 iu/l (12 King–Armstrong units/100 ml). On further investigation: the urine was seen to contain no bilirubin or urobilinogen; the reticulocyte count was 0.7%; 50% of the plasma bilirubin was unconjugated; a cholecystogram was normal.

(a) What was the diagnosis?
(b) Was a liver biopsy indicated?
(c) What additional test might assist in confirming the diagnosis?

Question 21.4

A woman aged 21 years was admitted with an inevitable abortion and a D and C was performed for necrotic infected retained products. Postoperatively the urine was red/black in colour. Investigations: Hb 8.2 g/dl (g/100 ml); white blood cell count 25 × 10^9/l (25 000/mm^3); neutrophils 87%; lymphocytes 13%; reticulocyte count 8%; indirect plasma bilirubin 94 μmol/l (5.5 mg/100 ml); platelets 75 × 10^9/l (75 000/mm^3).

(a) What were the diagnoses?
(b) What complications can occur?

Question 21.5

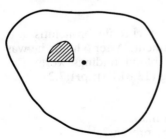

Figure 21.2

A 50-year-old man complaining of painless blurred vision for 24 hours is found to have this field defect in the right eye (*Figure 21.2*).

(*a*) How is the defect produced?
(*b*) What are the commonest causes?

Question 21.6 ✓

A man aged 27 years, height 206 cm with a high, arched palate and hyperextensible finger joints complained of distorted vision.

What urinary constituent should be measured to confirm or refute the diagnosis?

Question 21.7 ✓

During investigation of a megaloblastic anaemia 2.0 µg of radioactive vitamin B_{12} was given orally and 1000 µg of non-labelled vitamin B_{12} was given intramuscularly 1 hour later. Urine was collected for 48 hours and contained 11% of the labelled vitamin B_{12}.

What further investigations are indicated?

Question 21.8 ✓

After 2 years of continuous drug therapy a woman aged 27 years sought advice regarding constipation. Investigations: serum calcium 2.79 mmol/l (11.2 mg/100 ml); serum magnesium 1.1 mmol/l (2.6 mg/100 ml); ESR 17 mm in the first hour (Westergren); serum thyroxine 50 mmol/l (3.9 µg/100 ml); TSH 14 mU/l.

(*a*) What drug had this patient been taking?
(*b*) Name two other side-effects.

Question 21.9 ✓

A man aged 25 years was treated with lithium carbonate for a manic depressive neurosis for 18 months. For the latter 5 months of treatment nocturia was reported. Investigations: urine sterile; blood urea 4.5 mmol/l (22 mg/100 ml); serum electrolytes normal; overnight urine osmolarity 425 mmol/l; plasma lithium concentration 0.9–1.3 mmol/l.

(a) What biochemical abnormalities were present?
(b) Explain the nocturia.

Question 21.10 ✓

A 34-year-old male nurse who trained in the Navy complains of lassitude and more difficulty than usual in staying awake on night duty. Hb 182 g/l; haematocrit (PCV) 0.54; mean cell volume (MCV) 101 fl; RBC volume 30 ml/kg; serum iron 20 μmol/l; total iron binding capacity (TIBC) 60 μmol/l; ferritin 250 μg/l; red cell folate 125 μg/l; serum B_{12} 800 ng/l; AST (SGOT) 40 iu/l; ALT (SGPT) 46 iu/l.

Give two diagnoses.

Paper 22

Question 22.1 ✓

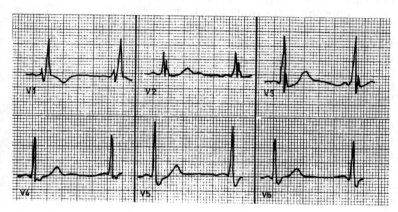

Figure 22.1

(*a*) What diagnoses are likely from the above chest leads (*Figure 22.1*)?

(*b*) Describe the abnormalities present.

(*c*) Name five possible causes.

Question 22.2 ✓

A man aged 45 years had an intermittent arthropathy for 10 years. He was found to have a Fredrichson's Type IV hyperlipoproteinaemia.

87

(*a*) What is the probable nature of the arthropathy?
(*b*) What are the two commonest presentations of this disorder?
(*c*) What are the biochemical features of Type IV hyperlipoproteinaemia and what is the inheritance?

Question 22.3 ✓

A woman aged 24 years with multiple ileoileal, ileocolic and
ileocutaneous fistulae due to Crohn's disease was treated for 2
months with total parenteral nutrition. From time to time she
developed paraesthesiae, weakness and had occasional convulsions. The following results of investigations were reported on
blood samples taken during an attack: blood urea 5.2 mmol/l
(33.5 mg/100 ml); serum calcium 2.57 mmol/l (10.3 mg/100 ml);
serum phosphate 0.43 mmol/l (1.3 mg/100 ml); serum albumin
34 g/l (3.4 g/100 ml); serum magnesium 0.95 mmol/l (2.28 mg/
100 ml); plasma sodium 139 mmol/l; plasma potassium 2.9 mmol/l;
plasma chloride 97 mmol/l; plasma bicarbonate 32 mmol/l; blood
glucose 11.3 mmol/l (201 mg/100 ml); plasma cholesterol 4.1 mmol/
(160 mg/100 ml); P_{O_2} 106 mmHg (14.1 kPa), P_{CO_2} 37 mmHg
(4.9 kPa); pH 7.49.

(*a*) What was the diagnosis?
(*b*) What was the probable cause in this woman?
(*c*) How may this be avoided?

Question 22.4 ✓

A woman aged 48 years presented with polydipsia and polyuria of
3 months' duration. Investigations: urine volume 5–8.5 l/day;
blood urea 5 mmol/l (30 mg/100 ml); mean of five measurements of
plasma osmolarity 285 mmol/l; following intramuscular vasopressin urine volume fell to 4.5 in 24 hours but polydipsia continued.

What was the diagnosis?

Question 22.5 ✓

A 66-year-old man complains of unsteadiness on his feet. He is
found to have impairment of deep pain sensation (squeezing the

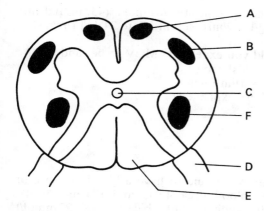

Figure 22.2

Achilles tendon) and also of proprioception in the toes but can feel the touch of cotton wool.

(*a*) Which of the pathways in *Figure 22.2* may be damaged and what is their name or names?
(*b*) Explain the findings.
(*c*) Suggest a likely cause and two alternatives.

Question 22.6 ✓

A 71-year-old man with a history of worsening nocturia presents with backache which prevents him from sleeping. Investigations: Hb 11.5 g/dl (g/100 ml); ESR 70 mm in the first hour (Westergren); serum calcium 2.3 mmol/l (9.2 mg/100 ml); serum phosphate 1.0 mmol/l (3.1 mg/100 ml); alkaline phosphatase 206 iu/l (29 King–Armstrong units/100 ml); total acid phosphatase 10.2 iu/l (5.6 King–Armstrong units/100 ml).

(*a*) What is the diagnosis?
(*b*) How may it be confirmed?

Question 22.7 ✓

A man with a known blind loop had the following results: Hb 10.7 g/dl (g/100 ml); reticulocyte count 2.2%; serum iron 12 µmol/l

(67 µg/100 ml); iron binding capacity 78 µmol/l (437 µg/100 ml); serum vitamin B_{12} 80 ng/l (pg/ml); serum folate 24 µg/l (ng/ml).

(*a*) In what range would you expect the MCV to be, and why?
(*b*) What will a Schilling test show?
(*c*) Comment upon the serum folate.
(*d*) How are these findings explained?

Question 22.8

A woman aged 25 years was found to have a blood pressure of 155/110. Investigations: blood urea 4.0 mmol/l (24 mg/100 ml); plasma potassium 3.0, sodium 140, bicarbonate 27 mmol/l (mEq/l); plasma aldosterone 155 pmol/l. She was treated with spironolactone 300 mg daily and in 18 days the blood pressure was 135/90 mmHg.

What was the diagnosis?

Question 22.9

An elderly woman with established cirrhosis and portosystemic encephalopathy deteriorated cerebrally despite a low-protein diet and neomycin 2 g daily. The dose of neomycin was trebled with improvement in cerebral function but 3 months later the patient developed diarrhoea. Investigations: Hb 10.2 g/dl (g/100 ml); MCV 115 fl (µm³); white blood cell count 4.5 × 10⁹/l (4500/mm³); alanine transaminase (ALT/SGPT) 65 iu/l; serum alkaline phosphatase 248 iu/l (35 King–Armstrong units/100 ml); serum albumin 39 g/l (3.9 g/100 ml); xylose excretion 13% excreted in 7 hours; faecal fat 49.3 mmol/day (14 g/day).

What are the probable diagnoses?

Question 22.10

A 31-year-old woman is unconscious following a major convulsion. Plasma sodium 111 mmol/l; potassium 4.2 mmol/l; urea

5.5 mmol/l; bicarbonate 18 mmol/l; glucose 4.2 mmol/l; calcium 2.5 mmol/l; albumin 42 g/l; serum osmolarity 234 mOsm/l; urine osmolarity 830 mOsm/l; urinary sodium concentration 113 mmol/l.

(a) Give three possible mechanisms of the hyponatraemia.
(b) Which is the most likely, and why?

Paper 23

Question 23.1

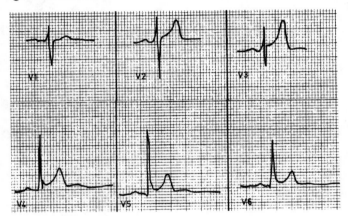

Figure 23.1

(a) What abnormalities are present in these chest leads (*Figure 23.1*)?

(b) What is the diagnosis?

(c) Would symptoms be present?

Question 23.2

A 50-year-old man with a 25-year history of abdominal pain has: blood urea 14.0 mmol/l (84 mg/100 ml); plasma sodium 135, potassium 3.0, bicarbonate 32 mmol/l (mEq/l); anion gap of 12.

92

(*a*) With what condition are the above findings compatible?
(*b*) What would one expect the urine pH to be?

Question 23.3 ✓

A woman aged 56 years was admitted to hospital following a haematemesis. Among investigations performed were the following: serum IgM 2.20 g/l (220 mg/100 ml); antimitochondrial antibodies present 1 in 60; urine pH range 6.7–7.5.

What was the diagnosis?

Question 23.4 ✓

A man aged 40 years had progressive back and pelvic girdle discomfort. Investigations: X-ray of spine—'cod fish' vertebrae; X-ray of abdomen—nephrocalcinosis of medullary distribution; urine pH 7.0–6.4; 3 days' faecal fat excretion 13.5 mmol/day (3.8 g/day); D-xylose absorption 1.1 g excreted in 5 hours after 5 g orally; blood urea 5.5 mmol/l (33 mg/100 ml); serum calcium 2.0 mmol/l (8 mg/100 ml); serum phosphate 1.4 mmol/l (4.3 mg/100 ml); serum albumin 41 g/l (4.1 g/100 ml); arterial pH 7.3.

(*a*) What were the diagnoses?
(*b*) What confirmatory test was indicated?

Question 23.5

A 50-year-old woman complains of difficulty in walking. On examination she has bilateral extensor plantar responses with loss of pain and temperature sensation on the right from just below the umbilicus downwards and over the left hemithorax in a narrow band below the nipple.

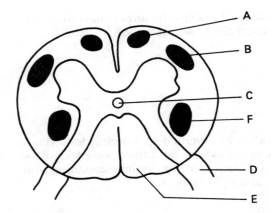

Figure 23.2

(a) Which of the pathways in *Figure 23.2* may be damaged and what is their name or names?
(b) Explain the findings.
(c) Suggest a cause and the exact site.

Question 23.6

A bottle-fed male baby aged 3 weeks was brought to Casualty in a state of collapse with a history of diarrhoea and vomiting for 1 day. Investigations: Hb 16 g/dl (g/100 ml); PCV 49%; blood urea 10 mmol/l (60 mg/100 ml); plasma sodium 150, potassium 3.5, bicarbonate 14 mmol/l (mEq/l).

(a) What diagnoses would be considered?
(b) What additional investigations should be performed?

Question 23.7

A patient with a megaloblastic marrow was treated with vitamin B_{12} when the Hb was 7.9 g/dl (g/100 ml). There was a 9% reticulocyte count on the fourth day. Despite continued twice-weekly intramuscular doses of vitamin B_{12} the haemoglobin failed to rise above 10 g/dl (g/100 ml).

(*a*) What was the most likely explanation?
(*b*) What other possibilities exist?

Question 23.8

A child aged 3 months who had been treated for neonatal hypoparathyroidism developed recurrent viral and *Candida* infections. Investigations: immunoglobulin concentrations normal for age; peripheral white blood cell count $3.8 \times 10^9/l$ (3800/mm^3), differential count polymorphs 89%, monocytes 1%, lymphocytes 10%. The majority of lymphocytes present bound fluorescent antigen. No spontaneous rosettes formed with sheep red blood cells. It was not possible to induce dinitrochlorobenzene skin sensitization.

(*a*) What was the diagnosis?
(*b*) What will a lymph node biopsy show?
(*c*) What is the treatment?

Question 23.9

A 26-year-old Indian woman had primary infertility. Plasma LH 26 iU/l (normal 5–10 iU/l); FSH 3 iU/l (normal 2–8 iU/l); testosterone 3.5 nmol/l (normal 1–2.1 nmol/l); prolactin 15 μg/l (normal 5–25 μg/l); urinary ketosteroids 30 μmol/24 h (normal).

(*a*) What is the diagnosis and why?
(*b*) How can it be confirmed?
(*c*) What serious rare complication can occur and why?

Question 23.10

A 30-year-old man attends the Outpatient Department routinely. Investigations show: Hb 100 g/l (10 g/dl); mean cell volume (MCV) 105 fl; white blood cell count 3.5×10^9; alkaline phosphatase 200 iu/l; γ-GT 35 iu/l; IgA 0.4 g/dl; urinary calcium excretion 1.8 mmol/24 h.

(*a*) What drug is he taking?
(*b*) List three physical findings.
(*c*) What other 'drug' could he be taking?

Paper 24

Question 24.1

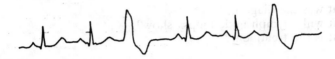

Figure 24.1

(a) What does this rhythm strip (*Figure 24.1*) show?
(b) State two possible underlying causes.

Question 24.2

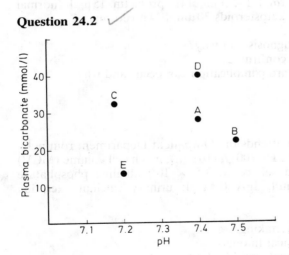

Figure 24.2

For each point A–E in *Figure 24.2* define the acid–base disturbance and give a possible clinical setting for the disturbance.

Question 24.3

A woman with diarrhoea mentioned symptoms of both hands. Investigations during an attack: serum calcium 2.19 mmol/l (8.76 mg/100 ml); phosphate 1.12 mmol/l (3.5 mg/100 ml); albumin 30 g/l (3.0 g/100 ml); arterial pH 7.39.

(*a*) What is the diagnosis?
(*b*) What should be measured for confirmation?
(*c*) In what type of patient does this develop?

Question 24.4

A 30-year-old woman complaining of recent weight gain has the following findings: glycosuria; creatinine clearance 159 ml/min; urea 2.5 mmol/l (15 mg/100 ml).

Suggest three explanations.

Question 24.5

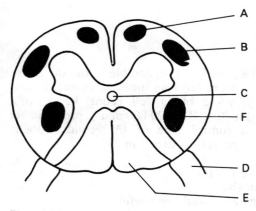

Figure 24.3

97

A 45-year-old man complains of bilateral shoulder pain worse at night for 2 months. He is found to have a band of reduced perception of pain and temperature around the thorax just above the nipples and wasting of the right arm. The tendon reflexes are absent from the right arm but those in the legs are present. The right plantar response is extensor and the left flexor.

(a) Which of the pathways in *Figure 24.3* may be damaged and what is their name or names?
(b) Explain the findings.
(c) Suggest a cause and the exact site.
(d) What further clinical sign may develop with lesions at this level?

Question 24.6

A 60-year-old man admitted for a hernia repair is found to have: plasma sodium 144, potassium 2.9, bicarbonate 35 mmol/l (mEq/l); blood urea 5.5 mmol/l (36 mg/100 ml).

(a) What metabolic derangement is present?
(b) Give six possible causes.

Question 24.7

A boy aged 8 years had a petechial rash and bled from the gums. He had recently suffered from German measles. Investigations: Hb 8.1 g/dl (g/100 ml); white blood cell count 4.5 × 10^9/l (4500/mm³); platelet count 20 × 10^9/l (20 000/mm³); prothrombin time 18 seconds with a control time of 13 seconds; rubella haemagglutination inhibition (HAI) titre 1 in 28.

(a) Comment upon these figures.
(b) What was the diagnosis?
(c) What other investigations would be useful?
(d) What is the treatment?

Question 24.8

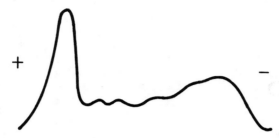

Figure 24.4

The above electrophoretic strip (*Figure 24.4*) was obtained from a patient with chronic disease.

(*a*) What abnormal features are shown?
(*b*) Suggest two diagnoses.

Question 24.9

A 17-year-old girl is brought to the Emergency Department because of abdominal pain, vomiting and shortness of breath. On examination there is peritonism, BP 80/40, heart rate 140/min, respiratory rate 36/min. Plasma sodium 105 mmol/l; potassium 5.4 mmol/l; urea 10 mmol/l (60 mg/100 ml).

(*a*) What two tests should be performed immediately?
(*b*) What is the diagnosis?
(*c*) Comment on the plasma sodium concentration.

Question 24.10

A Caucasian child aged 2 years has a mean cell volume (MCV) 110 fl, serum calcium 2.05 mmol/l, albumin 38 g/l.

(*a*) What is the most likely diagnosis?
(*b*) Explain the results.
(*c*) What HLA antigen is this child likely to have?
(*d*) Which cereals should be avoided?

Paper 25

Question 25.1

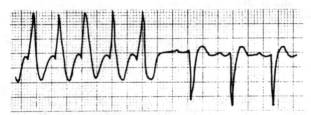

Figure 25.1

(*a*) What does the above trace (*Figure 25.1*) show?
(*b*) What simple manoeuvre changed the trace?
(*c*) What other measures are available?

Question 25.2

A thin 16-year-old girl has: serum calcium 1.97 mmol/l (7.9 mg/ 100 ml); serum inorganic phosphate 0.8 mmol/l (2.48 mg/100 ml); 25-hydroxyvitamin D_3 (25-OHD$_3$) 25% of standard reference sera.

(*a*) Suggest two diagnoses.
(*b*) What symptoms may such a patient have?

Question 25.3

A man with a long history of indigestion required admission to hospital. Investigations: urine pH 5.9; arterial pH 7.48; P_{CO_2} 41 mmHg (5.47 kPa).

(*a*) What is the acid–base disturbance?
(*b*) What was the underlying pathology?

Question 25.4

A man aged 51 years took medical advice because of two episodes of painless haematuria. The blood pressure was 175/122 mmHg. Investigations: urea 5.9 mmol/l (35 mg/100 ml); plasma electrolytes normal; urine microscopy—epithelial cells only; urine culture—sterile. The blood pressure was successfully treated. Two months later he felt unwell and was reinvestigated: urea 32.1 mmol/l (193 mg/100 ml); urine microscopy— many erythrocytes and white blood cells; no casts, urine culture sterile; IVP—poor opacification and dilatation of right renal pelvis, left kidney not demonstrated.

(*a*) What was the probable diagnosis?
(*b*) What urgent investigation was needed?
(*c*) Comment upon initial management.

Question 25.5

A 55-year-old merchant seaman complains of difficulty in walking. He has bilateral absent knee and ankle jerks and extensor plantar responses.

What is the differential diagnosis and what further investigations are needed?

Question 25.6

A woman aged 62 years with a controlled congestive heart failure developed an acutely tender knee joint. Investigations: Hb

12.9 g/dl (g/100 ml); white blood cell count 11.7 × 10^9/l (11 700/mm^3) with 78% neutrophils; blood urea 8.5 mmol/l (51 mg/100 ml); serum urate 0.65 mmol/l (10.8 mg/100 ml); ANF positive 1 in 5.

(a) What was the diagnosis?
(b) How may it be confirmed?
(c) What drug probably caused this condition?

Question 25.7 ✓

A woman aged 62 years presented with progressive jaundice. Investigations: bilirubin 402 μmol/l (23.5 mg/100 ml); alkaline phosphatase 873 iu/l (123 King–Armstrong units/100 ml); alanine transaminase (ALT/SGPT) 32 iu/l; γ-glutamyl transpeptidase 20 iu/l; Hb 11.5 g/dl (g/100 ml); ESR 43 mm in the first hour (Westergren); platelets 275 × 10^9/l (275 000/mm^3); prothrombin time 22 seconds, control 13 seconds; partial thromboplastin time 45 seconds, control 35 seconds; thromboplastin time 13 seconds, control 12 seconds; when normal plasma was added to the patient's plasma the PTT fell to 37 seconds.

(a) What was the overall diagnosis?
(b) What was the cause of the coagulation deficiency and which factors are affected?

Question 25.8 ✓

A woman aged 23 years presented with a 6-month history of arthropathy, adenopathy, Raynaud's phenomenon and dyspnoea. Investigations: ESR 69 mm in the first hour (Westergren); ANF positive 1:1024 with a speckled nuclear pattern on immuno-fluorescence; serum gamma globulin 70 g/l (7.0 g/100 ml); DNA binding less than 10%; CH50 97%. A high titre of antibody to ribonuclear protein was demonstrated.

What was the diagnosis?

Question 25.9

A woman aged 56 has lost 12 kg (26 lb) in weight over 2 years. Investigations show ESR 17 mm in 1 hour; Hb 10 g/dl; MCV 70 fl; albumin 37 g/l; alanine transaminase (SGPT) 20 iu/l; γ-glutamyl transpeptidase (GGT) 15 iu/l; alkaline phosphatase 250 iu/l; calcium 2.01 mmol/l (uncorrected).

(a) What operation did she undergo 10 years previously?
(b) What sequelae does she have and what other could she develop?

Question 25.10

A 22-year-old woman is brought to the Casualty Department complaining of severe abdominal pain. Plasma sodium 101 mmol/l; potassium 3.5 mmol/l; bicarbonate 8 mmol/l; urea 3.9 mmol/l; creatinine 200 μmol/l; amylase 700 u/l; white cell count 21×10^9/l.

(a) What is the diagnosis?
(b) What additional biochemical investigation was required?
(c) Explain all the abnormal results.

Paper 26

Question 26.1

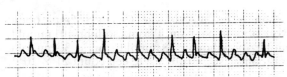

Figure 26.1

(*a*) What is this rhythm (*Figure 26.1*)?
(*b*) Suggest three common underlying causes and six rare ones.
(*c*) What is the treatment?

Question 26.2

A woman had a normal chest X-ray, FEV$_1$ of 3.9 and a PFR of 410 l/minute. The blood gases were: Po_2 59 mmHg (7.9 kPa); Pco_2 45 mmHg (6.0 kPa).

(*a*) What was her principal complaint?
(*b*) What was the major physical sign?
(*c*) What was the diagnosis?

Question 26.3

A Caucasian patient with Cushing's disease was treated by bilateral adrenalectomy. Three years later he returned to the clinic complaining of increasing deterioration of vision. Plasma adreno-corticotrophic hormone (ACTH) concentration was 4500 pg/ml.

(a) What was the diagnosis?
(b) What sign will probably be very obvious?
(c) What neurological signs could be expected to be found?
(d) What is the treatment?

Question 26.4

A man aged 65 years presented with haematuria and left loin pain. Investigations: urine—sterile; intravenous pyelogram (IVP)—mass arising from lower pole of left kidney with calyceal distortion; alkaline phosphatase 156 iu/l (22 King–Armstrong units/100 ml); isotope scan of liver—normal.

(a) What two further investigations should be performed?
(b) What was the diagnosis?

Question 26.5

CSF taken from a child who had had diplopia for 10 days contained the following: 0.17 cells × 10^9/l (170/mm^3) which were approximately half lymphocytes and half neutrophils; protein concentration 1.55 g/l (155 mg/100 ml); glucose 1.9 mmol/l (34 mg/100 ml); Gram stain of CSF—no organisms found.

(a) What was the probable diagnosis?
(b) What other investigations were needed?

Question 26.6

With some difficulty blood was obtained from a radial artery. The blood gases were Po_2 100 mmHg (13.3 kPa); Pco_2 24 mmHg (3.2 kPa); and pH was 7.48.

What was the diagnosis?

Question 26.7 ✓

A breast-fed male infant aged 3 days oozed blood persistently from the umbilical stump. Investigations: Hb 13.7 g/dl (g/100 ml); PCV 48%; platelets 155 × 10⁹/l (155 000/mm³); white blood cell count 13.5 × 10⁹/l (13 500/mm³), 60% neutrophils, 15% monocytes, 25% lymphocytes; bleeding time 4 minutes; prothrombin time 52 seconds with a control of 15 seconds; fibrinogen concentration 0.14 g/l (140 mg/100 ml).

(*a*) What was the diagnosis?
(*b*) What is the treatment?

Question 26.8 ✓

Three days after removal of a chronically rejected transplant kidney, blood taken at 08.00 hours had a serum cortisol concentration of 140 nmol/l (5.0 µg/100 ml). A dose of synthetic ACTH was given intramuscularly. Thirty minutes later the serum cortisol was 252 nmol/l (9 µg/100 ml).

What was the diagnosis?

Question 26.9 ✓

A woman aged 68 years with atrial fibrillation had been taking 0.25 mg digoxin daily for 9 years. At follow-up she reported anorexia, nausea and vomiting. Her pulse was 97 per minute. Investigations: blood urea 6.8 mmol/l (41 mg/100 ml); plasma creatinine 90 µmol/l (1.0 mg/100 ml); serum potassium 4.7 mmol/l (mEq/l); plasma digoxin 6 hours after the last dose 2.7 ng/ml.

(*a*) What was the diagnosis?
(*b*) What apparent discrepancy is there in the above figures?

Question 26.10 ✓

From a patient aged 47 years with severe psoriasis the following measurements were made: Hb 10.2 g/dl (g/100 ml); ESR 27 mm in

106

the first hour; white blood cell count $2.2 \times 10^9/l$ (2200/mm^3) with a normal differential count; MCV 117 fl (μm^3), MCHC 32 g/dl (g/100 ml); reticulocyte count 1%; serum B$_{12}$ 540 ng/l (pg/ml).

(*a*) How is the anaemia explained?
(*b*) How is it treated?
(*c*) What other complications may arise in such patients and how may they be minimized?

Paper 27

Question 27.1

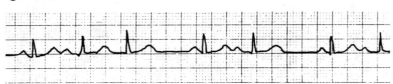

Figure 27.1

What does this rhythm strip (*Figure 27.1*) show?

Question 27.2

A known chronic bronchitic 55 years of age was admitted because of shortness of breath. Arterial blood gases (with the patient breathing air): Po_2 50 mmHg (6.6 kPa); Pco_2 62 mmHg (8.3 kPa); bicarbonate 18 mmol/l (mEq/l); pH 7.19.

(*a*) What metabolic abnormality do these results show?
(*b*) What three further blood tests are urgently required and why?

Question 27.3

A girl aged 18 months weighed 8 kg and was 75 cm high. Investigations: Hb 10.0 g/dl (g/100 ml); blood film—macrocytic; electrolytes normal; serum calcium 2.00 mmol/l (8.0 mg/100 ml);

total serum protein 50 g/l (5.0 g/100 ml); serum albumin 28 g/l (2.8 g/100 ml). After 5 g oral xylose the peak blood concentration of D-xylose was 19 mg/100 ml and the 5 h urine collection contained 0.8 g; bone age—approximately 10 months.

(*a*) What abnormalities were present?
(*b*) Under what two circumstances is the xylose absorption test invalid?
(*c*) What further investigations were necessary?

Question 27.4

In an adult, bilateral nephrocalcinosis was found in association with: osteoid border greater than 15 μm; urine calcium 2.1 mmol/day (84 mg/day); arterial pH 7.31; urinary pH 5.4.

What is the differential diagnosis?

Question 27.5

A 13-month-old child is febrile and vomiting. CSF shows: white cells 250/hpf (90% neutrophils); protein concentration 1.0 g/l (100 mg/100 ml); glucose 2.1 mmol/l (38 mg/100 ml); simultaneous blood glucose 6.2 mmol/l (111 mg/100 ml).

(*a*) What is the diagnosis?
(*b*) What further immediate tests should be performed on the CSF?
(*c*) What treatment is indicated?
(*d*) Why is the glucose low?
(*e*) What immunoglobulin will predominate in the CSF?

Question 27.6

A woman aged 66 years developed sudden back pain. Investigations: X-ray showed crush fracture of L2 vertebra; serum calcium 2.55 mmol/l (10.2 mg/100 ml); serum phosphate 1.2 mmol/l (3.7 mg/100 ml); serum albumin 40 g/l (4.0 g/100 ml); alkaline phosphatase 135 iu/l (19 King–Armstrong units/l); γ-glutamyl transpeptidase 15 iu/l; serum magnesium 0.9 mmol/l (2.2 mg/100 ml); urine calcium 4.47 mmol/day (190 mg/day).

(a) Assuming that no cancer was present, what was the diagnosis?
(b) How should it be confirmed?
(c) Name four conditions which may 'cause' this condition.

Question 27.7

A woman with vitiligo became anaemic. MCV 120 fl (μm³).

(a) What was the diagnosis?
(b) Name the three tests to prove the diagnosis.
(c) Suggest two immunological tests that are likely to be positive in this condition.

Question 27.8

The following were found in a baby 1 week old with intermediate genitalia: buccal smear chromatin positive; karyotype 46 XX; urinary ketosteroids 185 μmol/24 h (0.5 mg/24 h).

(a) Comment upon the results.
(b) What is the differential diagnosis of intermediate genitalia?
(c) What further investigations may be indicated?

Question 27.9

Figure 27.2 shows an echocardiogram from an adult.

What abnormality is present?

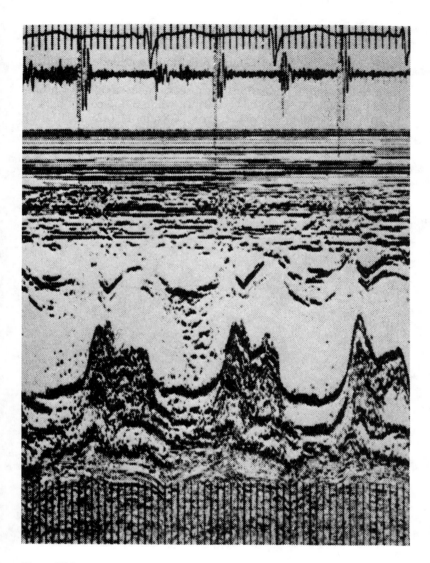

Figure 27.2

Question 27.10

A girl aged 17 years with stable renal failure attended her doctor for facial 'spots'. Tablets were prescribed. Ten days later she required hospital admission because of nausea and vomiting. Investigations: Hb 17.5 g/dl (g/100 ml); white blood cell count 17.5 × 10^9/l (17 5000/mm^3); blood urea 64.8 mmol/l (428 mg/100 ml); urine volume 190 ml in 6 hours; urine osmolarity 305 mmol/l.

(a) What was the diagnosis?
(b) Outline three steps in immediate management.
(c) What drug had she probably been given?

Paper 28

Question 28.1

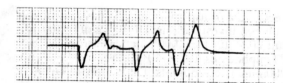

Figure 28.1

This rhythm strip (*Figure 28.1*) was taken from an ill man aged 19 years.

What does it show?

Question 28.2

Eight weeks after a successful renal transplant a man aged 29 years was admitted because of fever, cough and tachypnoea of 12 hours' duration. Investigations: chest X-ray showed fine granular opacities throughout both lung fields; Po_2 63 mmHg (8.4 kPa); Pco_2 31 mmHg (4.1 kPa); pH 7.5.

(*a*) What working diagnosis should be made?
(*b*) What investigations are essential?
(*c*) What is the treatment?

113

Question 28.3

Investigation of a breast-fed baby aged 4 days showed the following: plasma bilirubin 210 μmol/l (12.3 mg/100 ml); conjugated bilirubin 20 μmol/l (1.2 mg/100 ml); blood group A Rhesus positive; Coombs' test negative; Hb 13.0 g/dl (g/100 ml); serum aspartate transaminase (AST/SGOT) 20 iu/l; alkaline phosphatase 142 iu/l (20 King–Armstrong units/100 ml).

(a) What was the likely diagnosis?
(b) What is the differential diagnosis?
(c) What is the treatment?

Question 28.4

A patient who had received a transplant kidney 35 days previously developed a flu-like illness. Investigations: Hb 10.7 g/dl (g/100 ml); white blood cell count 20 × 10⁹/l (20 000/mm³), neutrophils 18 × 10⁹/l (18 000/mm³), lymphocytes 1.4 × 10⁹/l (1400/mm³), monocytes 0.2 × 10⁹/l (200/mm³), eosinophils 0.4 × 10⁹/l (400/mm³); platelets 100 × 10⁹/l (100 000/mm³); 24 hour urine volume 780 ml; creatinine clearance 43 ml/min; urine protein excretion 4.7 g/l.

(a) What was the likely diagnosis?
(b) Name six other features of this condition.

Question 28.5

A woman aged 49 years presented with earache, deafness and dribbling. A left lower motor neurone of the seventh nerve and left nerve deafness were present. There were vesicles on the ear, external auditory meatus and soft palate. Investigations: Hb 9.8 g/dl (g/100 ml); white blood cell count normal; blood film rouleaux present; ESR 102 mm in the first hour; electrolytes normal; alanine transaminase (ALT/SGPT) 60 iu/l; gamma globulin 61 g/l (6.1 g/100 ml).

(a) What was the cause of her symptoms?
(b) What was the cutaneous nerve supply of the area involved?
(c) What further investigations were indicated?

Question 28.6 ✓

A full-term 3.5 kg breast-fed male infant weighed 3.8 kg at 5 weeks. Investigations: bilirubin 72 μmol/l (4.2 mg/100 ml); aspartate transaminase (AST/SGOT) 10 iu/l; alkaline phosphatase 3400 iu/l (479 King–Armstrong units/100 ml). Urine was positive to Benedict's solution but negative to Clinistix.

(a) What was the diagnosis?
(b) How is the diagnosis confirmed?
(c) What is the treatment?
(d) What advice should be given to the parents?

Question 28.7 ✓

A 70-year-old man is found to have a platelet count of $1000 \times 10^9/l$ (1 000 000/mm^3).

What is the differential diagnosis?

Question 28.8 ✓

A talkative male aged 32 years presented with loss of libido of 2 years' duration. His weight had increased, gynaecomastia and soft testes were present. Investigations: plasma testosterone 6.5 nmol/l; plasma prolactin 247 μg/l. Thyroid-releasing factor (TRF) did not increase the prolactin concentration.

(a) What was the differential diagnosis?
(b) What additional investigations were needed?

testosterone low
prolactin ↑

Question 28.9 ✓

A patient aged 37 years underwent a cardiac procedure. Two months later the following were observed: resting heart rate 95/minute; slow increase in rate upon exercise; an increase in left ventricular end diastolic pressure and cardiac output without changing the rate upon increasing the venous return by raising the legs.

(a) What procedure had been performed?
(b) Explain the findings.

Question 28.10 ✓

A Caucasian woman of 19 years was found to have a blood pressure of 180/125 mmHg. IVP normal; peripheral venous renin 3490 pg ml^{-1}h^{-1}; blood urea 12 mmol/l (72 mg/100 ml); GFR 48 ml/min; urine microscopy no abnormality; proteinuria 1.9 g/day.

(*a*) What was the diagnosis?

She was successfully treated with oral diazoxide and frusemide. One week later the peripheral venous renin was found to have approximately doubled in concentration and the GFR had fallen to 33 ml/min.

(*b*) Comment upon the increase in the renin and the fall in GFR.
(*c*) Comment upon the drug treatment.

Paper 29

Question 29.1

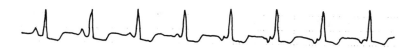

Figure 29.1

(*a*) What does this rhythm strip (*Figure 29.1*) show?
(*b*) What treatment is required?

Question 29.2

A woman aged 35 years was found to have a blood pressure of 165/105 mmHg. She complained of thirst, polyuria and muscle cramps. The plasma potassium was 2.5 mmol/l and arterial pH 7.49.

(*a*) What is the diagnosis?
(*b*) Explain the clinical findings.

Question 29.3

A 6-year-old Asian girl has a mean cell volume (MCV) of 108 fl, serum calcium 2.0 mmol/l, albumin 33 g/l.

What are the possible diagnoses and why?

Question 29.4 ✓

A 33-year-old single female insulin-dependent diabetic whose renal failure has been treated by hospital haemodialysis for 2 years complains of shortness of breath after 4 hours of a planned 6 h dialysis. Blood gases drawn from the fistula needle while breathing air: pH 7.56 ($[H^+]$ = 28 nmol/l), Pco_2 2.5 kPa (18 mmHg), Po_2 12.1 kPa (91 mmHg), HCO_3 19 mmol/l.

What is the diagnosis and why?

Question 29.5 ✓

A child aged 3 years received phenytoin and phenobarbitone because of epilepsy. The phenytoin level was 2 mg/l and the phenobarbitone level was 4.5 mg/l.

(a) Comment on these figures.
(b) What may be seen clinically?

Question 29.6 ✓

A girl aged 19 years was admitted after a suicide attempt. Initial blood gases were: Po_2 103 mmHg (13.7 kPa); Pco_2 29 mmHg (3.8 kPa); pH 7.48.

(a) What biochemical disturbance is present?
(b) What drug had the woman probably taken?
(c) What acid–base changes may occur later?

Question 29.7 ✓

An immigrant child aged 7 months was referred because the white blood cell count was found to be 17.0 × 10^9/l (17 000/mm³) and leukaemia was feared. Further investigations: platelet count 210 × 10^9/l (210 000/mm³); blood film—few myelocytes and myeloblasts, some nucleated red blood cells, marked poikilocytosis and target cells present; MCHC 26 g/dl (g/100 ml); MCV 57 fl (μm³); reticulocyte count 7%.

(*a*) What was the probable diagnosis?
(*b*) What physical signs were expected?
(*c*) What confirmatory investigation was needed?
(*d*) Name two characteristic X-ray appearances of this condition.

Question 29.8 ✓

A 30-year-old man being investigated for diarrhoea has an MCV of 115 fl (μm^3). Fluorescent studies upon material obtained at a jejunal biopsy showed a predominance of IgM-containing plasma cells. Serum IgM was 2.5 g/l (250 mg/100 ml) and IgA was not demonstrated.

(*a*) What was the probable diagnosis?
(*b*) Explain the findings.
(*c*) What HLA antigen would you expect this patient to possess?

Question 29.9 ✓

A 20-year-old man died suddenly while playing football. There was a 12-month history of palpitations. An ECG had shown ventricular ectopics and T-wave inversion in leads V1–3. An echocardiogram showed a dilated right ventricular cavity with dyskinesis and impaired contractility.

(*a*) What is the diagnosis?
(*b*) Suggest four other causes of sudden death in a man of this age.
(*c*) What were the post-mortem findings?

Question 29.10

A 38-year-old woman presents with a swollen neck. There is a family history of early death and her BP is 190/115 mmHg. Investigations show: corrected serum calcium 2.9 mmol/l (11.6 mg/100 ml); creatinine 130 μmol/l (1.5 mg/100 ml); resting calcitonin concentration normal; T_3 2.8 nmol/l (4.31 ng/ml); TSH 3 mU/l.

(*a*) What is the most likely diagnosis?
(*b*) What three further biochemical tests are required?
(*c*) How is this condition inherited?

Paper 30

Question 30.1 ✓

The following oxygen saturations were recorded in a patient aged 21 years:

Chamber	Oxygen saturation (%)
Superior vena cava	65
Right atrium	66
Right ventricle	67
Pulmonary artery	69
Left atrium	83
Left ventricle	75
Femoral artery	73

(a) What was the diagnosis?
(b) Should surgery be recommended?

Question 30.2 ✓

A woman aged 29 years had dyspepsia and haematuria. Investigations: Hb 10.0 g/dl (g/100 ml); MCV 68 fl; blood urea 5.2 mmol/l (31 mg/100 ml); serum calcium 2.95 mmol/l (11.8 mg/ 100 ml); serum albumin 41 g/l (4.1 g/100 ml); serum magnesium 1.2 mmol/l (2.9 mg/100 ml); serum phosphate 0.76 mmol/l (2.35 mg/100 ml); alkaline phosphatase 71 iu/l (10 King–Armstrong units/100 ml); serum urate 0.25 mmol/l (4.2 mg/100 ml); urine calcium excretion 8.6 mmol/day (345 mg/day); urine culture—*Escherichia coli*.

(*a*) What were the diagnoses?
(*b*) Name two radiological confirmatory investigations.
(*c*) Name a biochemical confirmatory test.

Question 30.3

A 4-day-old baby, birth weight 2.8 kg, was noted to have a convulsion. Investigations: blood glucose 1.7 mmol/l (30 mg/100 ml); serum calcium 2.0 mmol/l (8.0 mg/100 ml); prothrombin time 14 seconds with a control of 13 seconds; plasma sodium 135, potassium 4.0, bicarbonate 20 mmol/l (mEq/l); urea 4.1 mmol/l (35 mg/100 ml).

(*a*) What was the probable diagnosis?
(*b*) What further investigations should have been undertaken?

Question 30.4

A 16-year-old boy has an episode of renal colic. The urine is sterile but contains red cells 5000×10^6/l. The IVU shows bilateral radio-opaque calculi. Hexagonal crystals are seen in an early morning urine sample after acidification and cooling.

(*a*) Suggest three further tests.
(*b*) What is the diagnosis and treatment?

Question 30.5

A man aged 77 years had progressive hip joint discomfort for 2 years. Investigations: Hb 12.9 g/dl (g/100 ml); white blood cell count 4.9×10^9/l (4900/mm^3) with a normal differential; ESR 30 mm in the first hour (Westergren); serum calcium 2.6 mmol/l (10.4 mg/100 ml); serum phosphate 1.4 mmol/l (4.3 mg/100 ml); serum albumin 37 g/l (3.7 g/100 ml); alkaline phosphatase 212 iu/l (30 King–Armstrong units/100 ml); serum urate 0.46 mmol/l (7.7 mg/100 ml); urine calcium 8.3 mmol/24 hours (332 mg/24 hours); urine hydroxyproline excretion raised.

(*a*) What was the diagnosis?
(*b*) What is the explanation of the abnormal findings?
(*c*) What drugs are available to treat this condition?

Question 30.6

A patient with Fredrichson's Type IV hyperlipidaemia was treated with clofibrate and cholestyramine. He developed a venous thrombosis of the right calf and was given intravenous heparin for 48 hours followed by warfarin. On the third day a severe gastrointestinal haemorrhage occurred.

Why?

Question 30.7

A man aged 24 years presented with right upper abdominal quadrant pain, tenderness and fever. Investigations: urine—bilirubin present; plasma bilirubin 128 μmol/l (7.5 mg/100 ml); alkaline phosphatase 206 iu/l (29 King–Armstrong units/100 ml); alanine transaminase (SGPT) 35 iu/l; Hb 9.9 g/dl (g/100 ml); MCHC 38 g/dl (g/100 ml); MCV 83 fl (μm³); blood film—red blood cells smaller and darker than normal; Coombs' test negative; reticulocyte count 9.9%.

(*a*) What were the diagnoses?
(*b*) What additional history was necessary?
(*c*) What other physical signs would have been expected?

Question 30.8

A boy aged 3 years with severe combined immune deficiency received an ABO and HLA identical marrow transplant from a female donor. Female polymorphonuclear cells were seen in the peripheral blood 10 days after the transplant but at 18 days the boy developed diarrhoea with a macular eruption of the trunk and then face and hands. Aspartate transaminase (AST/SGOT) 180 iu/l; alanine transaminase (ALT/SGPT) 220 iu/l; bilirubin 85 μmol/l (4.6 mg/100 ml).

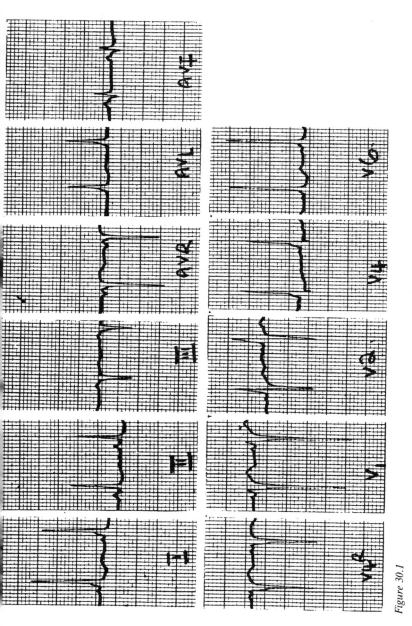

Figure 30.1

123

(*a*) What diagnosis must be considered likely?
(*b*) What preventative measures are now taken to avoid it?

Question 30.9

The ECG shown in *Figure 30.1* is from a 24-year-old man complaining of palpitations.

(*a*) List four abnormalities on the ECG.
(*b*) What is the exact diagnosis and defect?
(*c*) What are the dangers and what is the treatment?

Question 30.10

A 16-year-old boy has persistent bleeding 12 hours after a dental extraction. There is no family history. Investigations show: Hb 114 g/l; white blood count 9.8×10^9/l; platelets 400×10^9/l; prothrombin time 12.6 s (control 13.2 s); partial thromboplastin time (PTT) 86 s (control 42 s); bleeding time 12 min.

(*a*) What is the diagnosis?
(*b*) What is the defect?
(*c*) What is the treatment?

Answers and Discussion

Answer 1.1

This child had an atrial septal defect (ASD) with a left-to-right shunt. There was a step up in oxygen saturation in the right atrium when oxygen saturation is usually about 65–70% in this chamber. Because oxygenated blood was gaining access to the right heart, oxygen saturation in the right ventricle and pulmonary artery was much higher than usual.

Answer 1.2

(*a*) The agglutination of the red blood cells suggests that cold agglutinins were present. This finding occurs in more than 50% of patients with *Mycoplasma pneumoniae* infections. Leucocytosis is frequently absent.

(*b*) The diagnosis is substantiated by demonstrating:

 (*i*) a positive complement fixation test to *M. pneumoniae*;

 (*ii*) the presence of cold haemagglutinins.

(*c*) The treatment is tetracycline 2 g daily for 10 days.

Answer 1.3

She could have cirrhosis, nephrotic syndrome or congestive cardiac failure. The ascitic albumin level is that of a transudate— <25 g/l (2.5 mg/100 ml)—ascites being due to portal hypertension or hypoalbuminaemia.

Ascitic fluid with a high protein content (>25 g/l) is an exudate and occurs in association with malignancy, tuberculosis, pancreatitis, myxoedema or bacterial peritonitis. The latter may occur spontaneously in ascites in cirrhosis (alcohol-induced or otherwise).

Answer 1.4

Dehydration. He is oliguric but the high urine osmolarity, the urine/plasma (U/P) osmolar ratio of 2.37 (700 ÷ 295) and the low urinary sodium indicate normal renal response to fluid deprivation. The raised urea is a reflection upon the dehydration and in the presence of oliguria urea clearance falls. The serum osmolarity is at the upper limit of normal. Given adequate hydration the blood urea will return to normal.

Answer 1.5

(a) It was very probable that this patient had disseminated or multiple sclerosis (DS/MS). An increase in gamma globulin to 25% of the total without increase in the total protein content of the CSF is found in about 60% of patients with established disease. This increase in gamma globulin explains the abnormal colloidal gold curve. This increase in gamma globulin is mainly IgG in MS and the IgG:total protein ratio is often high (> 15%)

(b) In about 20–30% of patients with MS a high titre of measles antibodies in the CSF is found although the interpretation of this observation is unclear. Immunoelectrophoresis is carried out in specialized centres and shows oligoclonal bands of IgG not present in blood and therefore assumed to be synthesized intracerebrally.

Answer 1.6

(a) It is unlikely that a blood urea of 29 mmol/l (175 mg/100 ml) will produce persistent vomiting; a serum calcium of 3.8 mmol/l (13.5 mg/100 ml) is much more likely to be the cause.

(b) Primary hyperparathyroidism could explain all the abnormalities. If the vomiting has been severe enough, dehydration and pre-renal impairment could have occurred. Alternatively, hypercalcaemia may have led to hypercalcaemic nephropathy and renal impairment. However, one should consider a condition which may cause both hypercalcaemia and renal damage. Myeloma leads to hypercalcaemia via bone lesions and can depress renal function in a number of ways (e.g. myeloma kidney). Theoretically, sarcoid may cause both hypercalcaemia and depression of kidney function but renal sarcoid is rare.

Answer 1.7

(a) This woman had a low serum iron in the presence of a normal ferritin. This is a common but non-specific finding in ill people. It is seen in a variety of diseases as part of a response to 'inflammation' without any concomitant iron deficiency. An additional but probably not clinically important point is that serum iron has a diurnal variation, being higher in the morning than the evening.

(b) If doubt exists about the iron status, a bone marrow sample can be stained for iron stores or urinary iron excretion measured after a dose of parenteral desferrioxamine.

Answer 1.8

(a) This woman had Cushing's disease (pituitary-dependent bilateral adrenocortical hyperplasia due to excess pituitary production of ACTH). This is shown by the suppression of plasma cortisol (and hence the excessive ACTH) by dexamethasone.

(b) The disease may be treated at either the adrenal or pituitary level. Bilateral adrenalectomy followed by maintenance cortisone is very effective. The pituitary can be irradiated either externally or by an intrapituitary implant of yttrium-90. Metyrapone and/or aminoglutethimide, which interfere with cortisol synthesis, may be needed to supplement irradiation therapy or prior to bilateral adrenalectomy.

Answer 1.9

(a) Wiskott–Aldrich syndrome.

(b) Sex-linked recessive.

(c) Anaemia, thrombocytopenia, low serum IgM and IgG and a high IgA (normal ranges for a child of this age, 0.5–2.0, 5–14, 0.5–1.8 respectively). There was also a low T-cell count (normal

$500\text{--}1200 \times 10^3/l$). The B-cell count was normal ($250\text{--}110 \times 10^3/l$). (*d*) Supportive treatment with antibiotics, blood and platelet transfusions are of limited benefit. Bone marrow transplant is probably the treatment of choice if a suitable donor can be found. Splenectomy may help some patients.

(*e*) These patients cannot respond to polysaccharide antigens but can to protein antigens. This results in secondary defects in T-cell function.

Answer 1.10

(*a*) Hypertrophic obstructive cardiomyopathy (HOCM). The left ventricular systolic and diastolic pressures are raised (normal 100–140/4–10) and the increased diastolic pressure, due to 'stiff' muscle walls, is typical. Patients present with angina in the third or fourth decade and the majority of cases are familial with autosomal dominant inheritance. Aortic stenosis should also be considered but the ECG would probably show left ventricular hypertrophy or ischaemia or both.

(*b*) In HOCM echocardiography shows thickening of the left ventricle, most noticeably at the upper septal region. There is systolic anterior motion (SAM) of the anterior leaflet of the mitral valve on to the septum and delayed closure of the valve.

Answer 2.1

The pulmonary arterial pressure was greater than the systemic arterial pressure. There was a high right ventricular systolic pressure but no increased arterial oxygen saturation in that chamber. There was therefore a ventricular septal defect (VSD) with a balanced shunt and pulmonary hypertension—the Eisenmenger syndrome.

Answer 2.2

(*a*) These are typical findings in a patient with an acute exacerbation of chronic bronchitis. There was hypoxaemia, hypercapnia and acidosis.

(b) With resolution of the acute state the oxygen tension rises to about 70–90 mmHg (9.3–12.0 kPa), the carbon dioxide falls to about 50 mmHg (6.6 kPa) and the blood pH is usually within the normal range (a compensated respiratory acidosis).

Answer 2.3

(a) It is very probable from the history and raised IgM that this woman had primary biliary cirrhosis. Antimitochondrial antibodies are very suggestive and are found in 90% of cases. These antibodies are directed against the inner lining of the cristae of mitochondria but may not be cytotoxic *in vivo*.

(b) A liver biopsy will show mononuclear cell infiltration with accumulation into lymphoid follicles and bile duct injury and destruction.

Answer 2.4

(a) He had a kidney transplant 5 years ago. There is often significant proteinuria in these patients. The raised mean corpuscular volume (MCV) reflects azathioprine therapy, and the failure of plasma cortisol to rise after synthetic ACTH suggests long-continued prednisolone treatment. Lupus nephritis is treated with the same drugs.

The MCV gradually rises with continuous azathioprine treatment—in many patients who have received transplant kidneys 5 or more years previously, the MCV is above 100 fl (μm^3). Other complications of azathioprine include anaemia, leukaemia, agranulocytosis, thrombocytopenia and jaundice.

(b) Alport's syndrome—hereditary nephritis and nerve deafness sometimes accompanied by ocular abnormalities.

Answer 2.5

He may have either early poliomyelitis, non-paralytic or paralytic, or the Guillain–Barré syndrome. At an early stage the CSF findings of these two diseases can be very similar and the differentiation is clinical. If CSF were re-examined a week later, that from a poliomyelitis patient would have a pleocytosis and no further increase in protein, while CSF from a patient with Guillain–Barré syndrome would have no pleocytosis but the well-recognized increase in protein would be present. CSF culture might later grow the polio virus.

Answer 2.6

The most likely explanation of hyponatraemia, hypokalaemia and hypercalcaemia would be an oat cell tumour of a bronchus producing both ectopic ADH and a parathyroid hormone (PTH)-like peptide (e.g. osteoclast-activating factor—OAF). Many other tumours also have this potential ability. Oat cell tumours tend to produce ADH, and squamous cell tumours PTH-like substances, but there is not an absolute distinction between them.

Answer 2.7

(a) This woman had paroxysmal nocturnal haemoglobinuria.
(b) Blood and urine should be examined for free haemoglobin. The presentation and figures given in this example are characteristic of paroxysmal nocturnal haemoglobinuria.
(c) The definitive test is Ham's test. The red blood cells in paroxysmal nocturnal haemoglobinuria are more readily haemolysed in acidified serum than are normal cells. Although the condition carries the term nocturnal, episodes of haemolysis are not necessarily overnight and haemoglobinuria is not found in one-half of series of patients. The basic defect lies in the erythrocyte membrane which is sensitive to complement lysis although a specific defect has not been described.

Answer 2.8

(a) This man had raised serum cortisol concentrations at 09.00 and 24.00 hours and after attempted dexamethasone suppression. He therefore had either an adrenal tumour (Cushing's syndrome) or ectopic ACTH production. He did not have Cushing's disease (chromophobe or less frequently basophil, adenoma) because in this condition the ACTH feedback control while set at a supranormal level will be suppressed by dexamethasone.

(*b*) Weakness of the legs could be due to hypokalaemia (secondary to the renal effects of excess cortisol) or a proximal muscle myopathy (quite frequent in Cushing's syndrome). Spinal cord compression by metastases from an ACTH-producing tumour (e.g. of bronchus) is another possible cause of leg weakness.

Answer 2.9

(*a*) Seropositivity in a patient with rheumatoid arthritis indicates that rheumatoid factor is detectable in the patient's serum.

(*b*) Rheumatoid factor is a specific IgM and IgG antibody directed against the patient's own IgG (antigen). The rheumatoid factor is synthesized in plasma cells within the synovium of affected joints and is an auto-antibody. Why such patients' immunoglobulins become immunogenic and induce the production of auto-antibodies is unknown.

(*c*) The foot should be examined for the Babinski response. If it is positive (extensor plantar) the lesion lies at the level of the cervical portion of the spinal cord (where the long tracts may be compressed by osteophytes or subluxation) or at the internal capsule (suggesting a stroke in a man of this age). If there is no extensor plantar response, then further examination of the foot may show other signs of a peripheral neuropathy which can complicate rheumatoid arthritis.

Answer 2.10

(*a*) She has digoxin toxicity, either iatrogenic or a deliberate overdose. Blood should be taken for an urgent serum digoxin concentration.

(*b*) Digoxin inhibits the cellular Na-K-ATPase which normally maintains the intra- to extracellular concentration gradient for sodium and potassium.

(*c*) When life-threatening hypotension or arrhythmias occur, intravenous digoxin-specific antibody fragments (F_{ab}) should be given. Digoxin has a higher affinity for these synthetic antibodies than for the endogenous receptors. The antigen–antibody complex is water soluble and has a low molecular weight, permitting rapid elimination by glomerular filtration. Gastric lavage should be performed if there has been a recent deliberate overdose and activated charcoal left in the stomach. Cholestyramine or colestipol reduce absorption of any drug remaining in the gut lumen.

Answer 3.1

(a) This child has a VSD as shown by the step up in oxygenation at right ventricular level. There is a left-to-right shunt.
(b) The physical sign is a pansystolic murmur heard at the left sternal edge in the third and fourth intercostal space with or without a systolic thrill.

Answer 3.2

(a) The sweat sodium was equivocal (a level of less than 40 mmol/l is normal and more than 70 mmol/l is abnormal). The serum IgA was low (normal range 0.4–1.45 g/l for a child of this age); secretory IgA may well be low also.
(b) The sweat sodium estimation should be repeated.
(c) The diagnosis is selective IgA deficiency. Frequent respiratory infections are a recognized problem in such patients. There is no specific therapy; each respiratory episode is treated as required.

Answer 3.3

(a) These are the biochemical features of chronic active hepatitis. The piecemeal necrosis of the liver helps to differentiate the condition from primary biliary cirrhosis.
(b) The condition will respond, at least initially, to corticosteroids but there is a distinct probability of subsequent development of cirrhosis and perhaps portal hypertension and liver failure.

Answer 3.4

There was a renal artery stenosis of the kidney which was drained by catheter B. The urine volume and sodium excretion are decreased from that kidney while the excretion of urea and *para*-aminohippurate (PAH) is increased. These are the biochemical features of a functionally important renal artery stenosis. Because of the decreased blood flow in the kidney which is supplied by the stenosed artery there is 'more' time available for sodium reabsorption and also for excretion of urea, creatinine and exogenous substances such as PAH.

Answer 3.5

(*a*) Vessel J, the right anterior cerebral artery. Motor signs are present with or without cortical sensory loss.
(*b*) Apraxia occurs if the left anterior cerebral artery is affected.

Answer 3.6

Myelodysplasia. Iron deficiency anaemia is excluded by the presence of stainable iron and the marrow does not appear overtly depressed by the cytotoxic therapy. There are three myelodysplastic syndromes (refractory anaemias) distinguished by ringed sideroblasts, macrocytosis or the presence of blast cells. Myelodysplasia with ring sideroblasts is associated with severe anaemia (typically microcytic) but relative preservation of white cell and platelet numbers. Pelger cells are granulocytes with bilobed nuclei. Myeloma predisposes to myelodysplasia, particularly when alkylating agents have been given. This complication usually arises 3–10 years after the diagnosis of myeloma has been made.

Answer 3.7

(*a*) This patient had an iron deficiency anaemia as shown by the reduced MCV (microcytic cells), the reduced MCHC, the low serum iron and the increased iron binding capacity.
(*b*) Some anaemia (9–11 g/dl) is common in rheumatoid arthritic

patients and is usually normocytic and normochromic. Non-steroidal anti-inflammatory drugs cause mild but persistent blood loss, as may steroid treatment.

(c) In this patient a different analgesic was then used and the haemoglobin gradually rose to 11 g/dl. The anaemia was thereafter refractory to oral and intramuscular iron so it was considered that the residual anaemia was that associated with rheumatoid arthritis.

Answer 3.8

(a) This girl had pseudohypoparathyroidism. If the facies were normal the differential diagnosis would include idiopathic hypoparathyroidism.

(b) (i) Parathyroid hormone (PTH) assay shows the presence of PTH at a concentration appropriate to the degree of hypocalcaemia.

(ii) The hands should be X-rayed, as the metacarpals are shortened, especially the fourth and fifth.

(c) The face tends to be rounded and flat with a small bulbous nose and straight mouth; squints may be present.

(d) There is end-organ resistance to the effects of PTH and this may be partial or complete and affect one or all target tissues. In some patients neither phosphaturia nor increased urinary cyclic AMP (cAMP) is stimulated by PTH infusions (type I) and in others there is a marked rise in urinary cAMP but no phosphaturic effect (type II). Occasionally severe skeletal changes of hyperparathyroidism arise with osteitis fibrosa indicating skeletal but not renal sensitivity to PTH.

Answer 3.9

(a) This patient had rheumatoid arthritis.

(b) This disease is characterized by an arthropathy associated in many patients with a positive rheumatoid factor.

(c) These effusions are exudates as shown by their high albumin concentration. A low glucose and high lactic dehydrogenase (LDH) concentration are characteristic of rheumatoid effusions. The multinucleate cells are epithelioid cells and are characteristic of rheumatoid effusions. Degenerating polymorphs are also usually seen.

(*d*) The differential diagnosis of the pleural effusion includes malignancy and tuberculosis as both can be associated with low glucose levels in the fluid.

Answer 3.10

(*a*) He has irritable bowel syndrome. The tests of absorption are all normal and so was his sigmoidoscopy and barium enema. The symptoms described are typical.

(*b*) Treatment is frequently unsuccessful but bulking agents or antispasmodics may help and psychotherapy has also been shown to be beneficial.

Answer 4.1

This child had an ASD and pulmonary stenosis. The ASD was diagnosed by the step-up in oxygen saturation in the right atrium due to a left-to-right shunt. (The further step-up in oxygenation in the right ventricle is simply a measure of further mixing of the oxygenated blood from the left heart.) The pulmonary stenosis is shown by the high right ventricular pressure and normal pulmonary artery pressure. The systolic gradient was 41 mmHg which is well into the pathological range. Usually a pulmonary valve gradient is not regarded as significant unless it is more than 20 mmHg as there is a Venturi effect across the valve, giving rise to a small gradient.

Answer 4.2

(*a*) This man had an obstructive pattern of lung disease such as is found in chronic bronchitis.

(*b*) The FEV_1 (1.3 litres) and the FVC (2.5 litres) are much reduced. The FEV_1/FVC ratio is 52%. In normal people the ratio is 70–80%. FEV_1 is reduced because of high airways resistance. The low FVC is due to airways closing with limitation of expiration.

(*c*) If this trace were obtained when the patient had no exacerbation of chronic bronchitis the arterial pH would probably have been normal, but hypoxaemia and hypercapnia tend to persist.

Answer 4.3

(a) The diagnosis from these data is that of an active hepatitic process.
(b) The second group of data fits only one diagnosis—that of lupoid chronic active hepatitis. The presence of a high titre of antinuclear and antismooth muscle antibodies with a high serum gamma globulin (which is chiefly IgG) and the absence of hepatitis B antigen make the diagnosis. High titres of rubella and measles antibodies are found in some of these patients also.
(c) The prognosis is very variable: this hepatitis is almost always progressive to a cirrhosis but the severity of the jaundice and malaise varies and there may be acute exacerbations. Mortality is greatest in the first 2 years when the condition is most active. Steroids prolong life in the short term but side-effects may be troublesome. Azathioprine may permit reduction in steroid dose but most patients eventually die of hepatocellular failure with or without portal hypertension. This is an organ-specific auto-immune disease and may be associated with the sicca syndrome, subtotal jejunal villous atrophy, rheumatoid arthritis, scleroderma or CRST syndromes.

Answer 4.4

There was a large quantity of protein and glucose in the urine. The normal urine protein excretion is not more than 200 mg/day and normal glucose excretion measured by the oxidase method is 50–300 mg daily. This man was a diabetic and had developed nephrotic syndrome which was shown to be due to the development of the Kimmelstiel–Wilson lesion.

Answer 4.5

(a) Vessel I, the right middle cerebral artery.
(b) Aphasia occurs if the left middle cerebral artery is affected.

(c) Loss of proprioception is common (but not always present) and this impairs prognosis as it makes physiotherapy much more difficult.

Answer 4.6

(a) This man was hypocalcaemic with a raised alkaline phosphatase. These findings in this context suggest an inadequate diet and osteomalacia secondary to vitamin D deficiency. Renal function may be considered normal for his age.

(b) X-ray of the chest and pelvis of this man showed the pseudo-fractures of the scapulae and pubic rami. Hand X-rays showed erosions of the lateral borders of the middle phalanges of the ring and little fingers.

(c) Treatment involves vitamin D and provision of an adequate diet at home.

Answer 4.7

(a) Thalassaemia minor and pyridoxine-responsive anaemia are the two most common explanations of this apparently refractory iron deficiency anaemia.

(b) In both disorders serum iron should be measured and the bone marrow examined. In both, the plasma iron is high and the marrow contains increased iron stores. Thalassaemia is diagnosed by electrophoresis of the haemoglobin. The pyridoxine-responsive anaemia is diagnosed by the response to oral pyridoxine in doses of up to 200 mg orally daily.

There are two further diagnostic possibilities, both rare. Firstly, a sideroblastic anaemia may have a hypochromic blood film. Secondly, there is a condition of congenital absence of transferrin. Here iron absorption is supranormal and an excessive iron level is found in some tissues. The marrow is low in iron and the erythrocytes are hypochromic.

Answer 4.8

(a) This woman had hypothyroidism. Almost always, thyroid failure is associated with increased TSH levels, except in pituitary or hypothalamic hypothyroidism when TSH is absent from the serum. The fact that this woman responded with a very brisk increase in plasma TSH indicates that she had tertiary (or hypothalamic) hypothyroidism. In secondary (pituitary) hypothyroidism there is a subnormal response of the serum TSH to the intravenous administration of TRH.

(b) With evidence of abnormal hypothalamic function the possibility of intracranial disease and hyposecretion of other pituitary hormones should be considered. A history of post-partum haemorrhage or shock following pregnancy should be sought as anterior pituitary infarction (Sheehan's syndrome) is one of the commonest causes of this in women.

Answer 4.9

(a) This man has accelerated or malignant hypertension.

(b) Diabetes mellitus or polyarteritis nodosa (PAN) can cause a retinopathy and hypertension. Coincidental retinal vein thrombosis or a bleeding diathesis such as occurs in acute leukaemia could cause fresh haemorrhages.

(c) A fasting venous plasma glucose level of 7.8 mmol/l or more or a random glucose level of over 11.1 mmol/l is diagnostic of diabetes. A raised ESR, eosinophilia and proteinuria may suggest PAN which could be confirmed by a renal biopsy. Acute leukaemia should be obvious from the blood film which may also suggest lymphoproliferative disorders that can cause hyperviscosity. A bone marrow aspirate may be indicated.

Answer 4.10

(a) This nurse had liver cell damage, a haemolytic anaemia, raised serum IgM and a lymphocytosis with a neutropenia. Many of the lymphocytes were characteristic of infectious mononucleosis.

(c) Confirmation may be obtained by the heterophil antibody test (Paul–Bunnell) and by the demonstration of a rising titre of antibodies against the Epstein–Barr virus. All the abnormal laboratory findings quoted in this example may be found in a patient with infectious mononucleosis.

Answer 5.1

(*a*) This man had aortic stenosis. There was modest elevation of the right heart pressures and a marked systolic gradient of 68 mmHg across the aortic valve.
(*b*) The treatment is aortic valvular replacement.

Answer 5.2

(*a*) This spirogram is typical of restrictive lung disease.
(*b*) The FEV_1/FVC ratio is 3/3.5 × 100 = 86%. In health the FEV_1 should be at least 70–80% of the FVC.
(*c*) In a normal man aged 39 years the FEV_1 should be about 4.5 litres and the FVC 5.7 litres, giving a ratio of 79%. In this patient the ratio is supranormal. This is because the FVC is reduced but the FEV_1 is not proportionately reduced. The ratio therefore rises.

Answer 5.3

(*a*) Intrahepatic cholestatic jaundice gives rise to this pattern of enzyme and bilirubin increase and is often seen in association with hypersensitivity reactions involving the liver. The normal serum albumin indicates that this is an acute type of lesion. In some patients blood and hepatic eosinophilia may be found.
(*b*) The hepatic histology would show intact overall architecture with centrizonal bile stasis. Liver cells show patchy necrosis. The portal zones usually contain mononuclear cells and eosinophils. The bile ducts are of normal calibre.
(*c*) The most common cause of a sensitivity type cholestasis is chlorpromazine but it occurs in less than 0.5% of patients treated with this drug. Other phenothiazines may induce a similar hepatotoxicity. There are many other potential drugs in this category: they include chlorpropamide, sulphonamides, erythromycin estolate, nitrofurantoin, diphenylhydantoin and imipramine.

Answer 5.4

(*a*) He has nephrotic syndrome (fluid retention, hypo-albuminaemia and proteinuria). The fact that the latter is highly selective strongly suggests that this child had a minimal change glomerulonephritis. Children have a tendency to retain fluid within the abdomen as well as peripherally and ascites is not normally a feature of an adult with nephrotic syndrome.

(b) The treatment of choice is prednisolone with which a rapid cessation of the proteinuria usually occurs. An 8-week course of cyclophosphamide may produce prolonged remission in relapsing cases and help to reduce the steroid requirements.

(c) The characteristic course of minimal change glomerulonephritis is one of relapse and remission. Treatment almost certainly induces remission of the condition more rapidly than no treatment but the process may remit without any drugs.

Answer 5.5

Vessel C, the posterior cerebral artery. The visual defect is characteristic.

Answer 5.6

(a) (i) X-ray of the spine would show the 'bamboo changes' (calcification of the paraspinus ligaments with squaring of the vertebral bodies) and fusion of the sacro-iliac joints with surrounding osteosclerosis and osteoporosis.

(ii) Tissue typing would show HLA B27 in 85% of patients with ankylosing spondylitis. This antigen occurs in 14% of the general population.

(iii) An assessment of renal function is required. In this case the creatinine was 500 mmol/l and the creatinine clearance 11.5 ml/min.

(iv) A rectal biopsy should be performed and stained with Congo red to identify amyloid.

(v) An echocardiogram is necessary to look for evidence of aortic incompetence—the presence of which is suggested by the wide pulse pressure (90 mmHg)—or poor left ventricular function which may suggest cardiac amyloidosis.

(b) This man had ankylosing spondylitis with associated aortic incompetence and both rectal mucosal and renal amyloidosis. He required dialysis four months later.

Answer 5.7

(*a*) This child had acute lymphoblastic leukaemia (ALL). Infectious mononucleosis (Paul–Bunnell test) may produce similar clinical and blood changes.

(*b*) Remission can be achieved in up to 90% of patients and is induced with drugs such as vincristine, asparaginase and prednisolone for a period of 6 weeks. This is followed by maintenance therapy with courses of vincristine, methotrexate and prednisolone, together with intrathecal methotrexate and prophylactic CNS irradiation to prevent CNS relapse. Therapy is continued for at least 3 years from remission.

(*c*) The 5-year survival is no better than 50% and of these some may still be on therapy because of relapses.

(*d*) A relatively poor prognosis is indicated by male sex, age <2 years, white cell count >$20 \times 10^9/l$ at presentation, presence of mediastinal or central nervous system involvement.

Answer 5.8

(*a*) This man had a raised GFR, together with hypercalciuria and raised plasma phosphate. These are all features of active acromegaly and his symptoms also fit the condition.

(*b*) (*i*) Measurement of an elevated plasma growth hormone (normally less than 10 ng/ml while at rest and fasting) and demonstration of failure to suppress secretion (normally to below 5 ng/ml) during an oral glucose tolerance test.

(*ii*) CT scan of the pituitary fossa.

(*c*) One-third of patients notice a change in their features, one-third are noticed to have abnormal features incidentally by a doctor and one-third complain of symptoms, as in this example.

Answer 5.9

(*a*) A long systolic murmur following a myocardial infarction probably represents the development of mitral incompetence or a VSD. Either abnormality may be complicated by the development of bacterial endocarditis and this is associated with fever, anaemia, leucocytosis and haematuria (suggesting a glomerulonephritis).

(*b*) Six blood cultures should be taken in the 24 hours following the presumed diagnosis and high-dose parenteral penicillin treatment should be begun as soon as the cultures have been taken. Streptococci are the commonest organisms (30–50%), and are usually penicillin sensitive. *Staphylococcus aureus* is approximately half as common but if acquired in the community up to 80% of strains may be sensitive to benzyl penicillin. Echocardiography will differentiate between mitral incompetence and a VSD. Surgery may be needed early in the clinical course to excise infected tissue, to patch the VSD or replace the mitral valve, especially when *S. aureus* infection is present.

Answer 5.10

This child had combined sickle cell disease and thalassaemia. The positive metabisulphite test indicates the presence of HbS. However, target cells are not a feature of sickle-cell disease but are very frequently seen in thalassaemia. In sickle-cell disease some red blood cells have increased and some have decreased osmotic fragility. This child, who was of Mediterranean origin, had HbS, HbF and some HbA_2 on electrophoresis.

Answer 6.1

There was a sharp drop in pressure somewhere in the aorta. The most common cause is coarctation. However, this patient had hypercalcaemia and abnormal facies which are associated with supravalvular aortic stenosis. This was the diagnosis in this child.

Answer 6.2

(*a*) This is a restrictive pattern of lung disease (2.8/3.1 × 100 = 90%).
(*b*) Such a pattern is found in ankylosing spondylosis. There is no increased airways resistance but movements of the thoracic cage are restricted so the FVC is reduced and the ratio FEV_1/FVC is supranormal.
(*c*) About 90% of such patients possess HLA B27.

Answer 6.3

(*a*) This man was a chronic alcoholic. Such people have early morning nausea and vomiting and bouts of diarrhoea. The hypochloraemia, hypokalaemia and alkalosis are explained by losses of sodium, potassium, hydrogen and chloride ions in the vomitus (the approximate concentrations of these electrolytes in gastric juice is 50 mmol/l, 12 mmol/l, 50 mmol/l and 45 mmol/l respectively).

(*b*) The low blood urea is a reflection of the subnutritional state of alcoholics—wine and spirits contain only trivial quantities of protein and alcoholics need to spend available money on ethanol, not food.

Answer 6.4

(*a*) This patient had osteomalacia and chronic renal failure.

(*b*) The normal concentration of 25-OHD$_3$ indicates adequate dietary vitamin D and normal hepatic hydroxylation of vitamin D$_3$. The very low 1,25-$(OH)_2D_3$ and 24,25-$(OH)_2D_3$ indicate failure of hydroxylation of 25-OHD$_3$ which takes place in the kidney. Chronicity of the renal disease is implied by the development of 'renal osteomalacia' (renal osteodystrophy). The grossly raised parathyroid hormone level was due to hyperphosphataemia and hypocalcaemia which occur in chronic renal failure unless specific therapeutic measures are taken to control plasma phosphate levels with oral phosphate-binding agents.

(*c*) The serum phosphate will lie in the range of 2.0–4.0 mmol/l (6–13 mg/100 ml) or more. Serum urate is likely to be 0.5–0.7 mmol/l (8–12 mg/100 ml) or more. These figures reflect chronic renal failure and, despite the urate concentration, attacks of gout are rare.

Answer 6.5

Vessel D, the basilar artery. Occlusive strokes in this vessel are often fatal when presenting with coma.

Answer 6.6

    (*i*)   Congestive cardiac failure
    (*ii*) Nephrotic syndrome
    (*iii*) Hepatic cirrhosis.

The data show: reduced blood volume (normal for males 69 mg/kg bodyweight), raised renin and raised plasma aldosterone. Together these changes constitute secondary hyperaldosteronism which may occur in the above conditions. Raised plasma aldosterone might suggest Conn's syndrome (primary hyperaldosteronism) but the raised renin and reduced blood volume are not found in this condition. In secondary hyperaldosteronism, arterial hypovolaemia is considered to be the stimulus to renin production. Despite venous congestion in congestive heart failure, arterial hypovolaemia results from the falling cardiac output. Arterial volume may also be diminished due to hypo-albuminaemia resulting from proteinuria in nephrotic syndrome or from deficient albumin synthesis in cirrhosis.

Answer 6.7

(*a*) The MCV is elevated (the limit of normal is 100 fl). The serum vitamin B_{12} is very raised and target cells (these are erythrocytes which have a well-stained central area, then an intermediate pale zone and a well-stained periphery) are present. These three features strongly suggest the anaemia of chronic liver disease. The explanation for macrocytosis in the presence of a normoblastic bone marrow and ample B_{12} is unknown.
(*b*) The next step in investigation of this man would be to examine his liver function. Indicated tests include: serum albumin, alkaline phosphatase, alanine transaminase (ALT/SGPT), bilirubin, clotting studies and perhaps liver biopsy.

Answer 6.8

(*a*) This man had the carcinoid syndrome.
(*b*) The diagnosis was established by measuring the urinary excretion of 5-hydroxyindole acetic acid (5-HIAA). Normal 24 h excretion of 5-HIAA is about 2–10 mg; in the carcinoid syndrome usually more than 50 mg/day are excreted.

(c) Other features involve transient hypotension with attacks of flushing induced by taking alcohol, pulmonary stenosis (and hence right heart failure), reversible airways obstruction leading to wheezing, abdominal discomfort, borborygmi and diarrhoea, pellagra and photosensitive dermatitis.

(d) Cyproheptadine and methysergide may help the diarrhoea. Intravenous somatostatin may be of use before surgery and a long-acting synthetic analogue may soon be available.

Answer 6.9

(a) This man had a postinfarction ventricular aneurysm as shown by the persistent ST elevation over the left ventricular leads and the bulge on the lateral border of the enlarged heart. ST segment elevation persists in only 25% of postinfarction aneurysms.

(b) The aneurysm will appear as a segment which does not move (akinetic) or bulges out paradoxically during systole (dyskinetic). The diagnosis can usually be confirmed by echocardiography but angiography may be necessary and must be performed. Surgery is indicated if there is persistent heart failure, angina, uncontrollable ventricular arrhythmias or systemic emboli. Aneurysm resection is often combined with coronary bypass surgery.

Answer 6.10

(a) The blood urea was raised. A bicarbonate of 18 mmol/l is not unduly low for a child with diarrhoea and vomiting. A Hb of 10.2 g/dl (g/100 ml) is not unusual in a toddler. The platelet count was low and petechiae should suggest the diagnosis of meningococcal septicaemia.

(b) Low platelets and blood in the stools suggest haemolytic–uraemic syndrome.

(c) This is confirmed by a blood film showing burr cells and a raised reticulocyte count.

(d) The clinical course would probably be one of rapid deterioration: intravascular haemolysis, falling haemoglobin and rising blood urea with oliguria. The overall mortality is 5–20% and varies according to the underlying aetiology.

Answer 7.1

(*a*) There was a step-up in oxygen saturation at atrial level, indicating an ASD which was of the ostium primum type since this lesion is frequently found in patients with Down's syndrome. If all the figures were obtained via a right heart catheter the child would have an endocardial cushion defect since this lesion allows a catheter via the inferior vena cava (IVC) to be manipulated into all the heart chambers.

(*b*) This was a male child with Down's syndrome.

Answer 7.2

(*a*) There was a combined respiratory and metabolic acidosis with hypoxaemia.

(*b*) The infant was premature both in terms of gestational age and of birth weight, and the probable diagnosis was therefore respiratory distress syndrome. The incidence of major congenital abnormalities, such as congenital heart disease, tracheo-oesophageal fistula and diaphragmatic hernia, is higher in low birth weight babies and has to be considered. Inhalation of regurgitated stomach contents may give rise to similar problems.

(*c*) A chest X-ray is essential. Respiratory distress syndrome will be confirmed by the typical ground glass appearance with an air bronchogram. Diaphragmatic hernia will be obvious if present and the size, shape and position of the heart and of the degree of vascularity of the lungs may be diagnostically useful. Patchy consolidation due to inhalation will also be demonstrated.

Answer 7.3

(*a*) This patient had mild elevation of ALT, AST, alkaline phosphatase and bilirubin. The AST elevation reflected the myocardial infarction but the alkaline phosphatase, bilirubin and to a lesser extent the ALT represented liver damage. The most likely explanation of these abnormalities is venous congestion of the liver secondary to right heart failure.

(*b*) Treatment is the administration of a potent 'loop' diuretic and, if atrial fibrillation is present, digoxin is indicated. With the control of the heart failure in this patient liver discomfort disappeared and the liver function tests became normal in 3 days.

Answer 7.4

(a) She has haematuria of glomerular origin and probably has one of the following four nephritides: Berger's C3/IgA (recurrent haematuria), Henoch–Schönlein purpura, membranoproliferative glomerulonephritis (mesangiocapillary glomerulonephritis) or acute post-streptococcal nephritis. Berger's lesion is the only one of the four possibilities which usually has a normal GFR at presentation. It is also associated with minimal urinary protein loss and often with a raised serum IgA. The ASOT is normal (<200 Todd units).

(b) The history should be expanded to include recent infections. Berger's nephritis often occurs at the height of, or shortly after, an upper respiratory tract infection and acute post-streptococcal nephritis has a latent interval of about 10–14 days following a streptococcal infection of the throat or skin. Acute post-streptococcal nephritis is now uncommon in Western Europe. Henoch–Schönlein nephritis tends to follow joint, skin (rash on the buttocks and extremities) and gut lesions (abdominal pain and bleeding).

Answer 7.5

(a) Vessel F, the right posterior inferior cerebellar artery (PICA).
(b) This is the lateral medullary syndrome. Occlusion of the PICA results in ipsilateral Horner's syndrome and contralateral sensory loss below the neck in addition to vertigo and dysphagia.

Answer 7.6

(a) The calculated osmolarity is 320.4, based on the formula:

$2[Na^+] + 2[K^+] + urea + glucose$
Thus: 300 + 8 + 7.2 + 5.2 = 320.4 (all concentrations expressed in SI units)

(b) Either direct measurement of the plasma osmolarity is incorrect or the plasma sodium (which contributes chiefly to the plasma osmolarity) measurement is inaccurate. The above calculation is not valid if there is gross lipaemia or hyper-proteinaemia or following an infusion of mannitol. This may be because measurements of plasma sodium is inaccurate in these circumstances or due to osmotic activity or unmeasured substances.

Answer 7.7

This is an iron deficiency anaemia in a patient who had a treated B_{12} deficiency anaemia. The B_{12} deficiency is on the basis of an atrophic gastritis; these patients have an increased incidence of carcinoma of the stomach. Such tumours bleed and cause iron deficiency anaemias. The probable diagnosis was therefore carcinoma of the stomach, which occurs in approximately 4% of patients with pernicious anaemia.

Answer 7.8

(a) She is thyrotoxic—TSH is suppressed.
(b) There is hypercalcaemia and hyperphosphataemia with a raised alkaline phosphatase. This is due to increased bone turnover—hypercalcuria and increased urinary hydroxyproline also occur and if left uncorrected may result in osteoporosis. With treatment of the hyperthyroidism, hypercalcaemia ceases. If this does not occur, then an alternative explanation of the hypercalcaemia has to be found.

Answer 7.9

These findings are compatible with the diagnosis of rheumatic carditis. The elevated ASOT indicates a recent β-haemolytic streptococcal infection. The tachycardia and prolonged PR interval (normal not more than 0.2 s) substantiate a carditis.

These features are also compatible with a streptococcal infection in a patient with pre-existing heart block or on quinidine therapy.

Answer 7.10

(a) This pedigree is an X-linked recessive pattern.
(b) The marriage of two cousins in generation III has resulted in the unusual case of an affected (as opposed to carrier) female in generation IV.

(c) Haemophilia A, glucose-6-phosphate dehydrogenase deficiency, Duchenne muscular dystrophy and congenital ichthyosis are all X-linked recessive disorders.

Answer 8.1

(a) The data indicate pulmonary stenosis (high right ventricular pressure and low pulmonary artery pressure) and a VSD with a right-to-left shunt. These are two features of Fallot's tetralogy; the other two components—right ventricular hypertrophy and an over-riding aorta—are demonstrated by ECG and angiography.

(b) The postero-anterior (PA) chest X-ray showed:

(i) a small pulmonary artery due to low pulmonary artery pressure;

(ii) a 'boot-shaped' heart due to right ventricular hypertrophy;

(iii) oligaemic lung fields.

Answer 8.2

(a) This patient had hypoxaemia with a low normal Pco_2. Two conditions which produce these findings are moderate pulmonary thrombo-embolism and lobar pneumonia.

(b) A large area of lung is not available for oxygen transfer, hence the hypoxaemia. As the reserve capacity for CO_2 transport is greater, the Pco_2 is normal, or reduced if there is tachypnoea. The failure of the Po_2 to increase following approximate doubling of the inspired oxygen concentration is due to imbalance between perfusion and ventilation of the diseased area.

(c) A ventilation–perfusion (V–Q) scan should be performed. In lobar pneumonia there is reduced perfusion and no oxygenation (a matched ventilation–perfusion defect) and in pulmonary embolism there is oxygenation but no perfusion (mismatched defects).

Answer 8.3

(a) This man had disseminated intravascular coagulation (consumption coagulopathy—DIC). There was a low platelet count, plasma fibrinogen was low and there was a raised titre of fibrinogen degeneration products (consumed fibrinogen). As this man had recent urgent bowel surgery it must be presumed that he had a Gram-negative septicaemia and that the DIC was secondary to the infection.

(b) Obstetric problems (amniotic fluid embolism and retained products of conception), leukaemias and incompatible blood transfusions may all cause DIC. Rarer causes include fungal septicaemias, profound hypothermia, pulmonary emboli and extracorporeal shunts.

(c) The major complications are usually seen together: bleeding, hypotension from the 'shock' of septicaemia and varying degrees of renal impairment. Jaundice is not infrequent and worsens the prognosis.

Answer 8.4

(a) The three essential features of nephrotic syndrome are present: pitting oedema, 'heavy' proteinuria and hypo-albuminaemia. Raised plasma lipids are not essential for the diagnosis but are a common finding resulting from raised lipoprotein concentrations which occur due to a generalized increase in hepatic protein synthesis. The urine sodium is much reduced—16 mmol/24 h—due to avid sodium retention as a result of secondary hyperaldosteronism. Sodium is stored extravascular-ly together with water and constitutes the pitting oedema. The nephrotic syndrome is not a diagnosis *per se* but a biochemical state—the underlying diagnosis is made by determining the renal morphology.

(b) The urinary aldosterone will be raised to 2–4 times the upper limit of normal. The diminished circulating volume of nephrotic syndrome stimulates the renin–angiotensin axis and is one of the major factors causing diminished sodium excretion.

Answer 8.5

(a) This boy had Wilson's disease. The serum copper is in the normal range (14–22 μmol/l) and in patients with Wilson's disease the range is 1.6–17.6 μmol/l. A proportion of these patients go through a self-limiting phase of a Coombs' negative haemolytic anaemia with subclinical hepatic disease and subsequently present with neurological, psychiatric or renal tubular disease (amino-aciduria, glycosuria and increased clearance of urate—the acquired Fanconi syndrome). The urine copper in this boy was characteristically raised, the normal range being 15–78 μmol/24 h. (b) The serum ceruloplasmin should be measured and would be found to be <1.3 μmol/l when the normal range is 1.8–2.5 μmol/l. (c) The additional sign which is always present when the condition has progressed to the neurological stage is the Kayser–Fleischer ring located at the periphery of the cornea in Descemet's membrane.

Answer 8.6

He had myeloma causing the nephrotic syndrome and renal impairment. He has hypoalbuminaemia, hypercalcaemia, hyperlipidaemia, hyperuricaemia and renal impairment. The measured serum calcium must be corrected for the hypoalbuminaemia as the ionized fraction is greater under these circumstances. Hyperlipidaemia frequently accompanies hypoalbuminaemia, probably due to excessive hepatic lipoprotein synthesis. Renal function is reduced but not sufficiently to account for the raised urate which reflects excess turnover in reticuloendothelial malignancies.

Answer 8.7

(a) This patient had a moderately severe iron deficiency anaemia. All indices of circulating red blood cells are low as is the serum iron. The iron binding capacity is raised.
(b) The most likely cause would be secondary to heavy periods. Bleeding from the gut such as occurs from an ulcer is also common. Iron deficiency anaemia is quite frequent following pregnancies, especially if they occur at short intervals. In a normal pregnancy about 750 mg of iron may be lost by the mother. A poor diet often is a contributory factor to any of the above causes.

Answer 8.8

(a) These findings indicate the presence of diabetes insipidus. The patient lost 3.5 kg in 8 hours and urine osmolarity remained low. There was therefore polyuria due to the absence of ADH. A normal response to fluid deprivation for 8 hours is a weight loss of less than 0.5 kg bodyweight and a rise in urine osmolarity to 700–1000 mmol/l.

(b) This man was known to have anterior pituitary failure and with cortisol treatment his ability to excrete water improved (as is usual) and nocturia developed. In addition to anterior pituitary failure he had posterior pituitary failure, the features of which were masked by cortisol deficiency.

Answer 8.9

(a) The man had dextrocardia. This is one of the causes of right axis deviation. Progressive loss of the QRS complex in the chest leads occurs because the electrode is placed increasingly further away from the left ventricle. The QRS loss is pathognomonic. The country of origin of the patient was immaterial.

(b) The apex beat is palpable in the right chest.

(c) Associated conditions: situs inversus, Kartagener's syndrome (sinusitis, bronchiectasis, situs inversus and dextrocardia).

Answer 8.10

(a) This man had a hyperviscosity syndrome on the basis of a Waldenström's macroglobulinaemia.

(b) Serum should be electrophoresed to demonstrate the much increased immunoglobulin peak and the IgM concentration quantified.

(c) The fundi showed extremely dilated venules and multiple haemorrhages.

(d) Urgent plasmaphaeresis is indicated to restore consciousness and preserve vision. Subsequently, cytotoxic therapy is needed.

Answer 9.1

(a) The pulmonary artery wedge pressure was raised, which implies raised left atrial pressure. The left ventricular pressures were normal. The diagnosis was therefore pure mitral stenosis.

(b) The chest X-ray may show an enlarged left atrium and a small left ventricle. The pulmonary artery may be prominent.

Answer 9.2

This man had late-onset intrinsic asthma as shown by the reduced peak flow rate, the obstructive FEV_1/FVC ratio which partially responds to isoprenaline and the sputum eosinophils. A circulating eosinophilia may also be present.

Answer 9.3

The problem was one of hypo-albuminaemia with normal hepatic function and no proteinuria. This suggests either malabsorption or loss of protein from the gut lesion. Progressive anorexia is a common feature of carcinoma of the stomach and occasionally some of these tumours exude protein to an extent sufficient to cause hypo-albuminaemia.

Answer 9.4

(a) There is a hypokalaemic, hyperchloraemic acidosis.
(b) The figures are compatible with adult renal tubular acidosis (RTA type I) and can also be secondary to ureterosigmoidostomy or ingestion of carbonic anhydrase inhibitors. In RTA there is a failure to maintain the normal gradient of hydrogen ions across the distal renal tubules. Bicarbonate is therefore lost in the urine in excess and results in a systemic metabolic acidosis. The 'anion gap' left by the reduced bicarbonate is 'filled' by chloride ion. Normally sodium is exchanged for potassium or hydrogen ions in the distal renal tubules. In RTA there is insufficient hydrogen ion available and potassium is exchanged for sodium—hypokalaemia results. RTA type I may cause hypercalcuria and nephrocalcinosis. Nephrocalcinosis can itself cause medullary damage and hence RTA.

In ureterosigmoidostomy, chloride and hydrogen ions are well absorbed from the bowel with resulting hyperchloraemia and acidosis. Potassium is the major large bowel cation and is not reabsorbed to any extent.

Answer 9.5

(a) He has carcinoma of the prostate and an associated polymyositis. Very high concentrations of acid phophatase are associated with metastatic deposits from carcinoma of the prostate. Also elevated are serum alanine transaminase, lactic dehydrogenase and creatinine kinase. All these enzymes tend to be elevated in polymyositis. Often in polymyositis related to a malignancy the muscle disorder becomes apparent before the tumour is demonstrable. Of polymyositis in general, an underlying tumour is found in about 10–20% of patients.

(b) (i) Electromyography (EMG) of an affected muscle is indicated and will establish the diagnosis with certainty. The features expected to be found are spontaneous fibrillation, salvoes of repetitive potentials, and short duration of polyphasic potentials of low amplitude.

(ii) A muscle biopsy would show necrosis and phagocytosis of muscle fibres and interstitial and perivascular infiltration of inflammatory cells.

Answer 9.6

The blood urea is raised substantially while the plasma creatinine is just above the upper limit of normal.

(i) The commonest cause is a heavy protein load which occurs after a gut haemorrhage.

(ii) With a very high protein diet a similar difference between urea and creatinine may be found.

(iii) Large doses of steroids exert a catabolic effect and hence cause isolated urea elevation.

(iv) A similar difference between urea and creatinine may occur in a bilateral amputee with about 60% loss of GFR. In this circumstance the amount of creatinine formed is reduced as the body muscle mass is diminished.

(v) In the elderly the GFR falls to about 50% of its value in youth due to senile nephron loss. Muscle mass is reduced in old age and hence less creatinine is produced. The rise in creatinine due to the reduced GFR may therefore be less than expected.

Answer 9.7

This child either had haemophilia A (Factor VIII) deficiency or haemophilia B (Factor IX) deficiency (Christmas disease). He did not have a von Willebrand disease: in that condition the bleeding time is prolonged as well as the PTT.

To differentiate between haemophilia A and B, assays for specific factors must be conducted.

Answer 9.8

(*a*) This woman had panhypopituitarism as shown by subnormal levels of thyroxine, cortisol, glucose, ACTH, growth hormone and the failure of growth hormone to rise during deep sleep. The condition is also called Simmonds' disease. Following a severe postpartum haemorrhage the condition is known as Sheehan's syndrome.

(*b*) Symptoms and signs may be vague but also include premature wrinkling of the skin and pallor (normochromic anaemia) loss of scalp, axillary and pubic hair and a general loss of secondary sex characteristics with atrophy of the breasts and genitalia. There may be headaches and visual impairment (optic chiasmal compression). The physical signs include bradycardia and hypotension.

Answer 9.9

(*a*) The left renogram trace is normal but the right side shows a progressive rise in isotope activity and no excretion. This is the pattern seen when the kidney is obstructed.

(*b*) The obstruction must be relieved as soon as possible to avoid permanent renal damage. The most likely cause is a calculus and removal from the ureter by Dormie basket may be possible. Alternatively the obstruction can be relieved temporarily by percutaneous nephrostomy or double-J stent inserted cystoscopically pending further investigations.

(*c*) The exact nature and site of the obstruction must be defined. If a stone is present its biochemical composition must be established and measurements made of the serum calcium and phosphate, urinary calcium and amino acid electrophoretic pattern and the serum parathyroid hormone concentration.

Answer 9.10

This woman had scleroderma (progressive systemic sclerosis), affecting the hands and the oesophagus. The immunological investigations point to no specific diagnosis but the history is very suggestive of scleroderma. While Raynaud's phenomenon is a fairly common condition, scleroderma develops in less than 2% of women with this vasomotor instability. Anticentromere antibodies occur in the CREST variant of systemic sclerosis (calcinosis, Raynaud's phenomenon, oesophagitis, scleroderma and telangiectasia). The prognosis of this is better than for diffuse scleroderma.

Answer 10.1

(a) This child had pure pulmonary stenosis as shown by the pressure gradient between the right ventricle and the pulmonary artery. There was no shunt as there was no step-up in oxygen saturation in the right side of the heart.

(b) The chest X-ray may show an enlarged main pulmonary artery due to poststenotic dilatation.

Answer 10.2

(a) This patient had a diffusion defect such as would be seen in cryptogenic fibrosing alveolitis or emphysema. Before exercise, while the partial pressure of oxygen was normal, the partial pressure of carbon dioxide was subnormal. These patients have to hyperventilate to maintain a normal partial pressure of oxygen and in so doing 'wash out' carbon dioxide and the partial pressure of carbon dioxide becomes subnormal.

(b) During exercise, the demand for oxygen exceeds the ability of the lung to deliver oxygen and the partial pressure falls. With tachypnoea the wash-out effect upon carbon dioxide increases, the P_{CO_2} falls further and the patient becomes alkalotic.

(c) The transfer factor T_{co} (D_{co}) should be measured to confirm the diagnosis. It would be reduced by at least 50% of the predicted value in this case and would not rise with exercise. For diagnosis of the underlying pathology a transbronchial lung biopsy may be required.

Answer 10.3

(a) The most likely reason for the development of steatorrhoea was the reintroduction of gluten either by relaxing the diet or by accidentally taking gluten. The other possibility was the development of small bowel lymphomata or carcinoma as both of these occur more commonly in patients with coeliac disease.

(b) The diagnosis of gluten reintroduction is made by history. A detailed dietary history taken by a dietitian may be needed. A small bowel lymphoma is diagnosed by small bowel radiography and subsequent open biopsy.

Answer 10.4

(a) Chronic renal failure after the introduction of a low-protein diet, following a dialysis, in the presence of persistent vomiting or in severe liver failure and renal impairment.

(b) There is a discrepancy between the plasma creatinine (approximately equivalent to a GFR of 10–15 ml/min) and urea (very approximately equivalent to a GFR of about 30–40 ml/min). In chronic renal failure after the introduction of a low-protein diet, the GFR is unchanged but the protein, and hence urea load to be excreted, is reduced. Haemodialysis or peritoneal dialysis removes urea more efficiently than creatinine because urea has a lower molecular weight and is therefore more easily cleared.

In the presence of persistent vomiting from any cause, more urea than creatinine is lost in the vomitus. Urea diffuses into all body fluids more freely than does creatinine and hence it is more available for loss from the stomach. Persistent vomiting also means that protein absorption will not be occurring.

The urea/creatinine ratio is also reduced in severe liver failure due to hepatic inability to metabolize amino acids to urea. The actual blood figures would be lower than in this discussion, e.g. urea 2.1 (14 mg/100 ml) and creatinine 148 μmol/l (1.7 mg/100 ml).

Answer 10.5

The head circumference is normal for this age of child. Intracranial calcification could be due to:

(i)   toxoplasmosis;
(ii)   hyperparathyroidism;
(iii) tuberose sclerosis;
(iv)   Sturge–Weber syndrome.

Answer 10.6

(a) This man had a high serum iron and an almost fully saturated iron binding capacity. He was diabetic and had a raised ALT. This man had idiopathic haemochromatosis. There is almost no differential diagnosis from these findings. Transfusion haemosiderosis is excluded as the patient was previously well and haemosiderosis from prolonged iron therapy is very uncommon.

(b) The fully established clinical picture of haemochromatosis is a combination of liver disease, diabetes, heart disease and skin pigmentation. There is an increased chance of a primary hepatoma. Men are very much more frequently affected than women, who are protected by the loss of iron during menstruation.

Answer 10.7

This man had both microcytes and macrocytes in the circulation at the same time. The microcytes and the MCHC of 30 g/dl reflect a pre-existing iron deficiency anaemia as might have occurred from chronic blood loss from a duodenal ulcer. The macrocytes are explained because after an acute bleed reticulocytes and normoblasts are seen in the peripheral film and both are larger than mature erythrocytes.

Answer 10.8

The investigations in this acromegalic indicated that he had anterior pituitary failure—this is caused by progressive enlargement of an eosinophilic adenoma of the anterior lobe of the pituitary. Eventually the tumour led to a pituitary infarction and hence hypothyroidism, hypoandrogenism (normal plasma testosterone for men 9–24 mmol/l (0.320–1.0 μg/100 ml)), hypoadrenalism and the failure of growth hormone to rise under the stimulus of hypoglycaemia and TSH to increase after TRH.

Answer 10.9

(a) There is a tachycardia and the T waves are symmetrically peaked.

(b) This may be a normal trace taken from a person with a thin chest wall or it may be associated with early hyperkalaemia. One should not rely upon an ECG to diagnose hyperkalaemia as hyperkalaemic changes may only become apparent at a dangerously high plasma potassium concentration or may never develop before the onset of ventricular fibrillation. The sequential changes as potassium rises are tall T waves, prolonged PR interval, flattening and loss of P waves and QRS widening.

Answer 10.10

A: Normal serum (Forssman antibody).
B: Serum from a patient with serum sickness.
C: This patient had infectious mononucleosis—glandular fever (positive Paul–Bunnell test).

Answer 11.1

The pressures indicate mitral incompetence and mitral stenosis. The right heart pressures were raised as was the pulmonary artery wedge pressure. In health, left atrial pressure is equal to the left ventricular end diastolic pressure and also the pulmonary artery wedge pressure. In this patient the gradient across the mitral valve was 16 mmHg (25–9). In an adult a gradient of more than 5 mmHg is usually taken to be clinically significant.

Answer 11.2

(a) This curve was obtained from a healthy person.
(b) This patient had severe air trapping with consequent persistent hyperinflated lungs. The tidal volume (inner curve) is considerably larger than the normal and the maximum respiratory exertion (outer curve) is much distorted. These measurements were obtained from a patient with advanced interstitial pulmonary fibrosis.

Answer 11.3

The important point in this case is to appreciate that the ascites was not due to hepatocellular dysfunction. Ascites of liver origin is always associated with hypo-albuminaemia. The peak flow rate suggests no serious lung disease; the low blood pressure and soft heart sounds suggest constrictive pericarditis, which is a well-recognized cause of ascites.

Answer 11.4

(a) This patient has chronic renal failure with a GFR of 14 ml/min. (b) He was taking a 30 g protein diet—this explains the discrepancy between the urea and creatinine concentrations which would not be found in acute renal failure. In chronic renal failure hypocalcaemia is very frequent. The raised urate and phosphate are found in both acute and chronic renal failure but thorough management of the patient with chronic renal failure should involve near-normalization of plasma phosphate by the use of phosphate-binding agents ($Al_2 (OH)_3$ or $CaCO_3$). The hyperlipidaemia is slight evidence in favour of a chronic lesion as mild elevation of serum lipids is found in many of these patients. The haemoglobin is only slightly reduced, which argues against chronic renal disease, but there is no direct relationship between nitrogen retention and haemoglobin.

Answer 11.5

(a) α-Fetoprotein in serum is raised in many cases of neural tube defect (spina bifida or anencephaly). A more significant correlation exists between amniotic fluid levels of α-fetoprotein and such defects. The levels rise as pregnancy progresses and more definite results would be obtained at 16–18 weeks than at 11–12 weeks. (b) Ultrasound localization of the placenta and amniocentesis. A significantly raised amniotic α-fetoprotein makes a neural tube defect very likely and termination of the pregnancy should be offered. The highest correlation is found between α-fetoprotein and anencephaly. A meningocele may exist with little or no increase in α-fetoprotein. (c) The incidence of neural tube defects is 1:600 in London and 1:250 in South Wales. Where a woman has already had an affected baby the risk rises to 1:40.

Answer 11.6

(a) This patient had Type A lactic acidosis, that is, lactic acidosis and tissue anoxia (Type B is lactic acidosis without tissue anoxia).

(*b*) Type A is found in association with cardiogenic shock, endotoxaemia, left ventricular failure and very severe anaemias. Survival relates to the blood lactate concentration at presentation and for levels of 9 mmol/l or greater, mortality is over 80%.

(*c*) Drugs may cause Type B lactic acidosis—especially biguanides (phenformin and metformin) and parenteral nutrition with fructose, sorbitol, xylitol or ethanol. An overdose of methanol or salicylates also causes lactic acidosis.

The other causes of Type B lactic acidosis are considered as a group and cause metabolic disturbances. These include diabetes mellitus, liver failure, renal failure and leukaemias.

(*d*) Treatment involves correction of the underlying condition and administration of intravenous bicarbonate of which very large quantities may be required. This may result in serious problems of sodium overload.

Answer 11.7

(*a*) The presence of myeloblasts in the peripheral blood film suggests that the patient had developed acute myeloid (myeloblastic) leukaemia as a complication or extension of his original polycythaemia. This occurs in about 25% of patients with polycythaemia rubra vera.

(*b*) The bone marrow is hyperplastic, the majority of cells being myeloblasts. The anaemia is consequent upon the leukaemic cells 'crowding out' the erythrocyte precursors.

(*c*) The prognosis is very poor, the average duration of survival from the time of diagnosis of this complication being only months.

Answer 11.8

(*a*) This electrolyte picture is entirely compatible with a diagnosis of Addison's disease or chronic hypoadrenalism. Hyponatraemia occurs because there is insufficient mineralocorticoid activity to permit the kidney to retain sodium adequately. The urinary sodium excretion rises disproportionately to dietary sodium and hyponatraemia occurs. In an attempt to compensate, the kidney retains an 'excess' of potassium and mild hyperkalaemia develops. The blood urea is usually normal as there is no significant impairment of the GFR.

(b) Addison's disease is confirmed by demonstrating a failure of rise in plasma cortisol following injection of synthetic ACTH. This test may be performed by intramuscular or intravenous injection according to the local protocol and laboratory reference ranges. A three- to fivefold rise in cortisol is usually seen.

Answer 11.9

This is an example of a paced ECG. The pacing 'spikes' immediately precede the QRS complex, which is widened. This example was taken from a patient with a permanent pacemaker, the 'spike' from a temporary pacemaker being smaller.

Answer 11.10

(a) Autosomal dominant (AD). Children therefore have a 50% chance of inheritance of the condition.
(b) Polycystic kidney disease, Huntington's chorea, neurofibromatosis, congenital spherocytosis, multiple polyposis coli. All occur more often than 1 in 10 000 live births.

Answer 12.1

(a) This patient had a third-degree heart block and the wide complexes suggest that this is infranodal; there is complete dissociation between the P waves (atrial rate) and the QRS complexes (ventricular rate). T-wave inversion in this context does not necessarily imply ischaemic heart disease.
(b) An artificial pacemaker should be inserted.

Answer 12.2

(i) The low blood oxygen and the normal CO_2 concentration make this a Type I pattern of respiratory failure. This is most frequently seen in an acute asthmatic attack.
(ii) These blood gas concentrations are also compatible with 'shock', e.g. systemic hypotension before hypercapnia has developed.

Answer 12.3

(*a*) This woman had acute pancreatitis as shown by the hyperglycaemia, the hypocalcaemia and the presence of methaemalbuminaemia. The methaemalbuminaemia results from tryptic digestion of extravasated blood around the pancreas.

(*b*) Important additional investigations are the measurement of serum and urinary amylase and arterial pH. Increase in amylase may be transient and is not specific for pancreatitis as it is elevated in perforated ulcer and intestinal obstruction although the increases rarely approach the levels found in pancreatitis.

(*c*) An erect abdominal X-ray should be taken to aid exclusion of a perforated ulcer. If the woman survives, gallstones should be excluded. In Britain gallstones are found in 50–60% of cases of acute pancreatitis.

Answer 12.4

(*a*) The patient had nephrotic syndrome (NS).

(*b*) There had been a rapid decline in renal function with worsening of the nephrotic syndrome. In the presence of sterile urine it is probable that a renal vein thrombosis had occurred. This is an infrequent but recognized complication of nephrotic syndrome of any origin but is particularly frequent when NS is due to membranous or mesangiocapillary glomerulonephritis.

(*c*) Non-invasive methods such as high-resolution ultrasound scanning or computerized tomography may show the thrombus. Renal vein angiography may be required.

(*d*) Thrombolysis may be performed either from a peripheral venous injection or at the time of venography, according to the available thrombolysin and clinical opinion. Many people, however, would merely anticoagulate with heparin and then warfarin.

Answer 12.5

This patient most probably had a viral meningitis but very similar CSF findings are found in secondary syphilis although in syphilis the cell count is unlikely to be quite as high as quoted in this example. A rash may be found in both conditions. Syphilitic meningitis is uncommon although abnormal CSF findings are found in 50% of patients with untreated secondary syphilis.

Answer 12.6 ✓

This man had pyrophosphate arthropathy (pseudogout, chondro-calcinosis). While features of this man's investigations suggest gout, the weakly positive birefringence of the joint crystals makes the diagnosis of pseudogout. Joint crystals of uric acid have a strong negative birefringence while those of calcium pyrophosphate dihydrate possess weak positive birefringence. The serum urate in this man was only about the upper limit of normal for his age although compatible with the diagnosis of gout.

Answer 12.7 ✓

(*a*) This man had polycythaemia rubra vera as shown by the raised haemoglobin, PCV and white blood cell count.
(*b*) Confirmation of the diagnosis is by demonstrating a red blood cell count of about $7-8 \times 10^{12}/l$ and a raised red cell volume of about 40–50 ml/kg bodyweight (normal range 30 ml/kg bodyweight). The bone marrow is increased in extent and shows increased red blood cells, myeloid cells and megakaryocytes. Neutrophil alkaline phosphatase staining is increased. Marrow iron stores are depleted. Serum B_{12} is often markedly raised. Chronic bronchitis is the most common cause of secondary polycythaemia and should be excluded by clinical examination and lung function tests.
(*c*) Treatment includes venesection, ^{32}P irradiation of the bone marrow or cytotoxic drugs—chlorambucil or busulphan. Overall survival is the same for treatment with ^{32}P or chlorambucil but there is an increased incidence of acute leukaemia in chlorambucil-treated patients. Pruritis responds to chemotherapy of the disease and both H_1 and H_2 histamine blockers help.

Answer 12.8 ✓

(*a*) This woman had myxoedema presenting with a carpal tunnel syndrome (myxoedematous compression of the median nerve at the wrist). Constipation and deafness are also recognized features of myxoedema.
(*b*) Pernicious anaemia is a condition caused by anti-intrinsic factor antibodies and there is an overlap with thyroid disease

which may also be mediated immunologically (antithyroid antibodies).

(c) Other features of myxoedema include: mental and physical sluggishness, cold intolerance, hypothermia, weight gain, croaking voice, dry and rough skin which may be yellowish and has a generalized non-pitting thickening of subcutaneous tissue, dry and brittle hair, menorrhagia, delayed relaxation of the tendon jerks, bradycardia, angina pectoris, peripheral cyanosis and Raynaud's phenomenon, 'depression' ('myxoedema madness').

Answer 12.9

(a) There is a tachycardia, the rate being about 200/minute. Each QRS complex is approximately equal in dimensions and the width represents more than 0.12 second (three small squares at the standard 25 mm speed of ECG paper). The QRS complexes are abnormal and dissociated P waves are present. These are all features of a ventricular tachycardia.

(b) A diagnostic feature (not shown) would be the presence of 'capture beats'—normal beats found amongst the tachycardia beats.

Answer 12.10

(a) This is an audiogram from the right ear. The symbols [ ] represent bone conduction and the symbols o and x represent air conduction on the right and left sides respectively.

(b) The audiogram shows a wide bone–air gap in auditory acuity (i.e. conductive hearing loss).

(c) The patient has polyarteritis nodosa (PAN) with a serous otitis media (a rare but well-documented complication). Virtually all organ systems may be affected by PAN and death usually results from renal, cardiac or respiratory complications.

Answer 13.1

(a) There are retrograde P waves present and the rate is 45/second. In addition there is ST depression. This was therefore a junctional bradycardia.

(*b*) This may be seen in digoxin toxicity which may also induce sinus bradycardia, AV block, ventricular ectopic beats and ventricular tachycardia. In this case sinus rhythm returned upon reducing the dose of digoxin.

Answer 13.2

This patient should have the following measurements:

(*i*) Sweat sodium.

(*ii*) The plasma level of α_1-antitrypsin

In patients with cystic fibrosis the concentration of sodium and chloride in the sweat is more than 70 mmol/l (mEq/l) (normal less than 40 mmol/l).

Levels of α_1-antitrypsin activity below 40% of normal are associated with the early development of emphysema, recurrent chest infections and further lung damage. α_1-Antitrypsin inhibits neutrophil elastase, normally released around inflammatory foci. Unimpeded, neutrophil elastase destroys tissues, the most vulnerable being the elastic connective tissue of the lung and liver. Prenatal diagnosis by chorionic villous sampling is possible at 12 weeks gestation and may help in genetic counselling.

Answer 13.3

(*a*) This case was an example of the Zollinger–Ellison syndrome (non-beta cell tumour of the pancreas). A basal secretion of 17 mmol/h of hydrogen ions is very high (normal basal H^+ secretion 0.5–5.0 mmol/h) and no increase follows pentagastrin injection as the patient's condition is due to excess endogenous gastrin production.

(*b*) Plasma gastrin can be assayed by a radioimmunoassay and fasting concentrations may be 25 times above normal and do not suppress following intravenous secretin challenge.

(*c*) The Zollinger–Ellison syndrome may be associated with functioning adenomas of the parathyroids and pituitary gland— Werner's syndrome or multiple endocrine adenomatosis type I (MEA I). Eighty per cent of gastrinomas are malignant.

Answer 13.4

A rise in blood urea of 16.8 mmol/l (101 mg/100 ml) in 24 hours is very rapid. Possible causes include:

(*i*) Gastrointestinal haemorrhage in a patient with chronic renal failure (e.g. a failing renal transplant after the administration of high-dose steroids).

(*ii*) This change may occur in a patient with septicaemia being treated with high-dose steroids for a rejection episode.

(*iii*) A laboratory error should also be suspected.

Answer 13.5

(*a*) Dependent oedema, hypo-albuminaemia and hypercholesterolaemia strongly suggest the presence of a nephrotic syndrome. With the reduced creatinine clearance it is highly probable that the glomeruli will show obvious damage when examined microscopically.

(*b*) The past history of this woman is typical of that of familial Mediterranean fever (FMF). At least 30% of patients with this condition develop renal amyloid disease which was demonstrated in this patient.

(*c*) The major drugs of use in nephrotic syndrome are spironolactone (to ameliorate secondary hyperaldosteronism) and a 'loop' diuretic. The former must be used with care when renal impairment is present.

Colchicine is of value in preventing the attacks of abdominal pain in FMF and may also prevent the development or progression of amyloid disease.

Answer 13.6

(*a*) The patient was unconscious and the blood glucose by calculation from the plasma osmolarity, sodium, potassium and urea was 29.6 mmol/l. Plasma osmolarity can be calculated by using the formula:

$$2[Na^+] + 2[K^+] + urea + glucose \text{ (all concentrations in SI units)}.$$

In this case the calculation is $300 + 9.8 + 13.6 + 29.6 = 353$.

(*b*) He has diabetes and tuberculous meningitis. The 6-week history of headache followed by coma in an Asian immigrant together with high CSF protein make the diagnosis of tuberculous meningitis a serious possibility. Ziehl–Neelsen staining of the CSF confirmed the diagnosis.

(*c*) The very high serum osmolarity is due to the high concentration of glucose and the hypernatraemia. The raised urea is a measure of dehydration consequent upon an osmotic diuresis and the diuretic, glucose, contributes to the raised urinary osmolarity.

Answer 13.7

(*a*) This is a leuco-erythroblastic blood picture as shown by the presence of white blood cell precursors and nucleated red blood cells in the peripheral blood.

(*b*) Confirmation is obtained by examining a stained smear of bone marrow aspirate.

(*c*) The disease may be associated with bony deposits from cancer of the breast, bronchus, stomach or prostate. It is also found in myelofibrosis, chronic myeloid leukaemia, myeloma, polycythaemia rubra vera, tuberculous infiltration of the bone marrow, sarcoidosis and osteopetrosis (Albers–Schönberg marble bone disease).

Answer 13.8

(*a*) This was a lag type curve because the highest glucose concentration was found at 30 minutes and the concentration then fell below usual levels at 60 and 90 minutes. The insulin response is slow proportional to the blood glucose concentration and subsequently is 'excessive'.

(*b*) A lag curve may be found:

(*i*) in post-gastrectomy and post-gastrojejunostomy patients in whom the glucose enters the small gut more rapidly than usual with consequent more rapid absorption.

(*ii*) in very severe liver disease, thought to be due to decreased glycogenesis.

(*iii*) occasionally in thyrotoxicosis, presumably secondary to very rapid glucose absorption.

(*iv*) in apparently normal people—reactive hypoglycaemia.

Answer 13.9

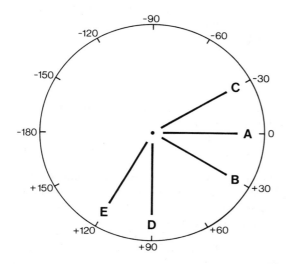

Figure 31.1

The answers are shown in *Figure 31.1*.

Answer 13.10

(*a*) Turner's syndrome. The basal LH and FSH levels are high and the oestradiol low suggesting gonadal dysgenesis. The murmur is probably due to coarctation of the aorta. Osteoporosis occurs due to oestrogen deficiency.

(*b*) Chromosome analysis. This shows a karyotype of 45 XO in the majority of cases of Turner's syndrome but mosaicism, partial deletions and ring chromosomes also occur and these modify the clinical manifestations. Turner's syndrome is the commonest chromosomal cause of osteoporosis.

Answer 14.1

(*a*) The ST segment is elevated in V2–V6 with deep Q waves in the same leads.

(*b*) This is the ECG of an acute extensive anterior transmural myocardial infarction.

(*c*) Predisposing factors include hyperlipidaemia, hypertension, use of the contraceptive pill, diabetes mellitus, cigarette smoking and a positive family history.

Answer 14.2

(*a*) There is a restrictive pattern of lung function (both FEV_1 and FVC reduced) and the ratio $FEV_1/FVC=85\%$. There is hypoxaemia and a reduced transfer factor.

(*b*) The diagnosis was an acute farmer's lung or extrinsic allergic alveolitis.

(*c*) The condition develops in some people 4–8 hours after inhalation of spores of *Micropolyspora faeni*, a thermophilic actinomycete found in mouldy hay. (There is very frequently a history of exposure to mouldy hay.)

(*d*) The disease is mediated by a Type III (Arthus) reaction. Circulating preformed antibody (not IgE) reacts with the inhaled antigen in the lungs, producing high concentrations of local immune complexes which cause complement activation and local inflammation.

(*e*) Treatment of the acute phase is with prednisolone. Long-term treatment is by the avoidance of mouldy hay and hence spores or, if that is not feasible, the use of a respirator while handling the hay.

Answer 14.3

These findings could occur in:

(*a*) coeliac disease, post-gastroenteritis and disaccharidase deficiency.

(*b*) coeliac disease, dermatitis herpetiformis, Zollinger–Ellison syndrome and in some cases of tropical sprue.

Answer 14.4

This was a spurious hyperkalaemia or pseudohyperkalaemia. The commonest cause is the blood sample having been left too long before centrifugation. Under these conditions red cell potassium leaks into the plasma, leading to falsely high readings. A similar situation exists in myeloproliferative disorders in which leakage of potassium from white blood cells can lead to hyperkalaemia in the plasma in a few minutes when white cell counts are very high. A rarer cause is 'familial pseudohyperkalaemia' in which abnormal cation transport across the red blood cell membrane results in potassium efflux over a few hours in blood stored at room temperature. This does not happen if the blood is kept at 37°C until the time of assay for potassium.

This woman is unlikely to have renal failure because hyperkalaemia in these patients is associated with acidosis and the plasma phosphate is very frequently raised. The data would fit the condition of hypoaldosteronism but this is a very rare disease.

Answer 14.5

(a) This patient had cerebral lupus. The high DNA binding (normal less than 25 U/ml; Amersham) indicates a high titre of antibodies against double-stranded DNA. The low C3 suggests complement consumption implying active systemic lupus erythematosus (SLE). The lymphocytopenia is frequently found in active lupus and very frequently in cerebral lupus. There are no characteristic features of the EEG in this condition, particularly in the absence of any focal sign. Up to 40% of patients with SLE develop organic psychiatric disease.

(b) Opinions differ regarding treatment. If there is no clinical evidence of disease elsewhere the patient may only require sedation during the neurotic phase. Other physicians would use steroids with sedatives. If there were focal neurological disease then steroids would be essential.

Answer 14.6

(a) This is Fredrichson's Type III hyperlipoproteinaemia. In addition to the abnormal cholesterol and triglyceride concentrations there are high levels of intermediate density and very low density lipoprotein (IDL and VLDL) and low concentrations of high density and low density lipoproteins (HDL and LDL).

(b) The defect is reduced catabolism of IDL and VLDL in the liver because of an abnormality of their apoprotein E (apo E) component—one of the constituents of these complexes. There is genetic polymorphism for apo E and patients with type III hyperlipoproteinaemia have the phenotype apo E 2/2. This occurs in approximately 1% of the population but another abnormality of lipid metabolism must coexist to result in clinical disease, impaired carbohydrate tolerance and hyperuricaemia.

(c) It is usually associated with the early onset of atherosclerosis (cardiovascular and peripheral vascular disease), xanthomata (cutaneous planar and tuberous), impaired carbohydrate tolerance and hyperuricaemia.

(d) Type III hyperlipoproteinaemia responds well to prolonged cholestyramine. Restriction of dietary cholesterol and saturated fats is also usually recommended. Clofibrate and bezafibrate may also have a role.

Answer 14.7

(a) This child had thrombocytopenic purpura (TCP). Further investigation would show prolonged bleeding time and increased capillary fragility. The bone marrow would show an excess of early forms of megakaryocytes which stain badly and scanty platelet budding. The condition may be idiopathic or occur 7–10 days after a viral illness—the commonest associations being infectious mononucleosis, mumps and rubella.

(b) TCP is usually self limiting and when the platelet count is $> 50 \times 10^9/l$ treatment is usually withheld. When the platelet count is $20 \times 10^9/l$ high-dose steroids should be given to suppress antiplatelet antibodies in view of the danger of bleeding (e.g. intracerebral). When the platelet count is $20–50 \times 10^9/l$ a therapeutic trial of steroids may be felt to be justified as long-lasting remissions may occur after short courses of treatment.

(c) In those few patients who relapse following prednisolone withdrawal, the liver and spleen should be scanned after intravenous administration of radio-labelled platelets. This may demonstrate the principal site of destruction. If this is the spleen, splenectomy will probably cure or ameliorate the condition.

Answer 14.8

(a) It was highly probable that this man had an oat cell carcinoma of the lung producing ectopic ACTH and hence much-increased (usually 2–10 times normal) plasma concentrations of cortisol. The renal effects of cortisol are sodium retention and compensatory excessive potassium loss. The hypokalaemia leads to an intravascular alkalosis (serum bicarbonate 33 mmol/l in this man). The glycosuria is explained by the diabetogenic effect of cortisol.

(b) A chest X-ray showed a mass at the right hilum and the urine contained ten times the normal 24 h excretion of 17-hydroxycorticosteroids, both before and after the administration of metyrapone and dexamethasone.

(c) The prognosis is very poor as an oat cell lung tumour is highly malignant and resistant to therapy. Those patients who have biochemical abnormalities at presentation frequently only have weeks to live.

Answer 14.9

(a) There is a posterior pericardial effusion as indicated in *Figure 31.2* on page 174. (ALMV, anterior leaflet of the mitral valve).
(b) A globular heart.

Answer 14.10

(a) This patient had renal osteodystrophy.
(b) He returned with hypercalcaemia and the reduced alkaline phosphatase gave evidence of healing of the bone disease.
(c) Before the administration of vitamin D analogues, the plasma phosphate concentration should have been reduced to < 2.0 mmol/l by the use of oral phosphate-binding agents (aluminium hydroxide capsules or calcium carbonate tablets). Alfacalcidol is 1-hydroxycholecalciferol and only requires 25-hydroxylation in the liver before becoming the active agent 1,25-dihydroxy-cholcalciferol. If vitamin D is given in renal impairment very high doses are needed. The follow-up interval was too great; the patient should have been seen at 2–3-weekly intervals to measure plasma calcium and to reduce the dose of vitamin D accordingly. Such a large dose as this would probably be necessary for only a very short time.
(d) Periarticular and vascular calcification may be demonstrated due to the solubility product for calcium phosphate having been exceeded.

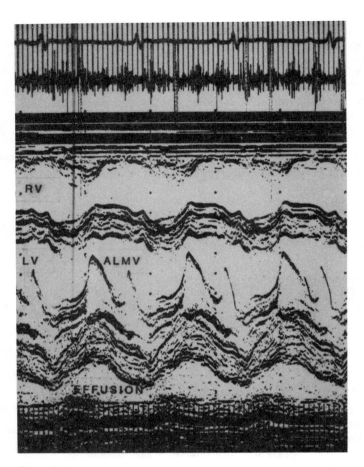

Figure 31.2

Answer 15.1

The first two complexes are normal; there are then four different beats. The four abnormal beats are regular and are supraventricular in origin. The P wave is buried in the T wave of the preceding complex and the QRS is different, implying aberrant conduction. As there are more than three consecutive extrasystoles, by definition this constitutes a tachycardia. The diagnosis is therefore supraventricular tachycardia with aberrant conduction.

174

Answer 15.2

There are only two possibilities: either there was an error in measuring the electrolytes or the blood taken for these investigations had been inadvertently diluted. Such a dilution occurs if the venous blood sample is taken from the same vein into which dextrose is being infused.

Answer 15.3

(a) Gaucher's disease.
(b) The adult form (chronic non-neuropathic) occurs in 1 in 2500 births in Ashkenazi Jews and typically presents with bony pain, avascular necrosis of the femoral head and pathological fractures. Recurrent abdominal pain is from splenic infarcts and from distension due to the splenomegaly. Grey-brown pigmentation of the forehead, hands and pre-tibial region occurs.
(c) A platelet count should be performed as thrombocytopenia may cause troublesome bleeding. This may be an indication for splenectomy as may painful abdominal distension. The bone marrow appearances are diagnostic and non-prostatic acid phosphatase is typically raised.

Answer 15.4

(a) She has chronic renal failure and hypertension. The sterile pyuria, microcytic anaemia and social background suggest analgesic abuse and analgesic nephropathy. Similar results could be found with urinary tuberculosis. A transitional cell carcinoma of the right renal pelvis may have developed (a rare late complication of analgesic abuse).
(b) Urine should be sent for cytological examination and early morning samples for Ziehl–Neelsen staining and culture for acid-fast bacilli.

Answer 15.5

(a) There was haemodilution, hyperkalaemia and respiratory acidosis. The haemodilution is consequent upon the inhalation and absorption of water across the alveoli. This is characteristic of fresh-water drowning. Respiratory acidosis occurs following inhalation of either fresh or salt water. Hyperkalaemia is a feature of both. Therefore this man died of fresh-water drowning.

(b) Immediately before a fresh-water death, ventricular fibrillation is the usual arrhythmia; after sea water, asystole.

Answer 15.6

(a) This man had hyperosmolar non-ketotic diabetic coma (HNC) as shown by the grossly elevated blood glucose, the hypernatraemia and the absence of ketones.

(b) The osmolarity by calculation was 393 mmol/l ($2 \times (Na + K)$ + urea and glucose—all measured in mmol/l).

(c) Patients with HNC are severely dehydrated with marked hypernatraemia and hypokalaemia. Relatively larger quantities of potassium are needed than in a patient with ketoacidosis and relatively smaller doses of insulin.

Despite the severe dehydration, fluid replacement should be less rapid than in ketoacidosis. This reduces the risk of cerebral oedema and allows serum osmolarity to fall to normal gradually. Because of the danger of arterial thrombosis, prophylactic heparin should be given, either subcutaneously or intravenously. Thiazides and diazoxide are both diabetogenic and apparently act as initiating factors.

Answer 15.7

(a) This man has myeloma.

(b) The raised MCV is due to folate deficiency as the rapidly dividing neoplastic cells utilize all available folate. Hypercatabolism also accounts for the hyperuricaemia and contributes to the hypoalbuminaemia. Hypercalcaemia is due to osteoclast overactivity resulting from local or circulating stimulant factors. Bence-Jones proteinuria (λ and $\varkappa$ chains in the urine) and hypercalcaemia impair renal function.

(c) The most significant adverse prognostic factors are anaemia (Hb <7.5 g/dl), renal impairment and restricted physical activity due to malaise. Hypercalcaemia is a less powerful predictor. The 2-year prognosis ranges from 10% to 75%.

(d) Melphalan and cyclophosphamide are most commonly used, either continuously or in intermittent high dose.

Answer 15.8

The most likely explanation of these figures in Western Europe would be amyloid disease of the so-called secondary type. Gut motility disturbances and malabsorption are common features of amyloid. Renal amyloid causes impairment of function and proteinuria (accounting for 10% of cases of nephrotic syndrome in the over-60s age group). Howell–Jolly bodies are a feature of hyposplenism which may occur in amyloid and bleeding diatheses due to factor X (and sometimes IX) deficiency and is a rare complication. Malabsorption may cause generalized vitamin K-dependent clotting factor deficiency.

Answer 15.9

(a) Dubin–Johnson syndrome. Patients are often asymptomatic but may have right upper quadrant pain, malaise and easy fatiguability. The gallbladder is typically not shown on oral cholecystograms. Urinary excretion of coproporphyrin I and III is in the ratio quoted.
(b) Autosomal recessive. Heterozygotes have intermediate coprophyrin I to III excretion ratios.
(c) A BSP (bromsulphthalein) retention test shows typical changes with early rapid clearance of this organic anion at 45 min followed by a rise at 90 min to levels greater than those at 45 min. There are now very few clinical indications for this test and severe anaphylactic reactions can occur.

Answer 15.10

(a) Gastroenteritis leading to dehydration and pre-renal renal impairment although the urea would probably be higher unless she has eaten nothing for several days.
(b) Addison's disease due to failure to absorb oral steroid therapy should be strongly considered. This could be deliberate omission of treatment, vomiting of ingested tablets or relative corticosteroid deficiency in the face of intercurrent illness.
(c) Liver failure (secondary to alcoholism or overdose of paracetamol or other hepatotoxin); renal replacement therapy leads to major psychological morbidity. Long-term azathioprine

may also be hepatotoxic.

(d) Emergency treatment of hyperglycaemia—too much insulin and insufficient intravenous sodium chloride. Steroid therapy may lead to diabetes in transplant recipients.

Answer 16.1

(a) This rhythm is atrial fibrillation as shown by the absence of P waves and the total irregularity of the QRS complexes.

(b) The most common causes are ischaemic heart disease and hyperthyroidism. Other causes include rheumatic heart disease, cardiomyopathy, constrictive pericarditis, acute fevers, post-thoracotomy, infiltration of the pericardium with tumours and pulmonary embolism. In addition a congenital form and an idiopathic or 'lone' form are described. If there is a predisposing cause atrial fibrillation is more likely to occur with advancing age.

Answer 16.2

(a) She has a phaeochromocytoma. The plasma noradrenaline, urinary metanephrines and 4-hydroxy-3-methoxymandelic acid (HMMA) or vanillylmandelic acid (VMA) are all elevated. The raised blood sugar and plasma potassium concentrations reflect excessive adrenergic activity. Similar results are also found after clonidine withdrawal. Raised VMA may be found in patients taking reserpine, guanethidine, α-methyldopa and phenothiazines because excretion products of these drugs interfere with the assay.

(b) Episodic severe pounding headaches associated with bouts of sweating, palpitations and anxiety attacks are commonly described (>50% of cases). Less frequently, tremor, nausea and vomiting, chest or abdominal pain and weight loss occur.

(c) CT scanning can detect tumours in the adrenals as small as 1 cm in diameter. Isotope scanning using ^{131}I meta-iodobenzyl-guanidine (MIBG) may be more sensitive and can also identify multifocal or metastatic tumours. Ten per cent of adrenal phaeochromocytomas are bilateral and 10% are malignant—these complications are more common in familial cases.

Answer 16.3

(a) α_1-Antitrypsin is deficient and the patient is homozygous for the protease inhibitor (Pi) ZZ gene.

(b) His activity will be approximately 15% of normal. Concentrations of 40% or more are required for health. Other genetic combinations and their percentage of normal activities are: PiMS (80%), PiMZ (60%), PiSS (60%), PiSZ (40%).

(c) In Northern Europe, 6% of the population are heterozygous for S (PiMS) and 4% for Z (PiMZ), making an overall frequency of 1 in 10 for the carriage of a deficiency gene.

(d) Liver transplant results in conversion to the genotype of the donor. Other diseases treated by liver transplant include primary liver tumours, primary biliary cirrhosis, Wilson's disease, Budd–Chiari syndrome and biliary atresia.

Answer 16.4

(a) Hyporeninaemic hypoaldosteronism. He is markedly acidotic and hyperkalaemic, disproportionately so for the level of renal function.

(b) Aldosterone concentrations are inappropriately low for the degree of hyperkalaemia. The condition is probably under-diagnosed; 50% of cases are diabetic and arterial disease is common. Hyporeninaemic hypoaldosteronism may result from reduced sensitivity of the renal stretch receptors due to arteriolar wall rigidity, insulin deficiency and autonomic neuropathy.

(c) Fludrocortisone in doses of up to 1.0 mg/day is the treatment and this may have to be combined with a thiazide or 'loop' diuretic to compensate for fluid retention.

Answer 16.5

(a) The raised cholesterol and LDL with the normal concentration of triglycerides make this a Type IIa of the Fredrichson and WHO classifications of hyperlipidaemia.

(b) Xanthomata may well be found.

(c) Nothing will occur. Serum from patients with Type IIa hyperlipidaemia does not become lactescent upon storage. VLDL cause lactescence and chylomicrons float to the surface leaving a clear subnatant.

Answer 16.6

The two most likely compounds are either paracetamol (acetaminophen) or carbon tetrachloride as both may produce combined renal and hepatic failure. A third possibility is phenol or one of its derivatives. Glycerol poisoning may produce a similar picture but with both these latter compounds death is likely to occur before 4 days.

Answer 16.7

This child had kala-azar (leishmaniasis). The diagnosis was made by finding Leishman–Donovan bodies in the bone marrow. The features of bleeding, weight loss, enlarged abdomen (liver and spleen), anaemia (haemolytic), leucopenia with lymphocytosis and greatly raised IgG are all characteristic of the condition.

Answer 16.8

He has Bruton's agammaglobulinaemia.

All tests of the cellular immune response are normal, as is the circulating lymphocyte count. The diagnosis is made by demonstrating that very little immunoglobulin is present. Serum IgG is rarely above 10% mean normal adult concentration and IgA and IgM are less than 1% of mean normal adult concentrations.

Note that despite repeated infections, peripheral lymph nodes and tonsils are hypoplastic and may be absent.

Answer 16.9

(a) Neural tube defects give raised levels of α-fetoprotein but they are also found in primary hepatoma.
(b) Although investigation of the embryo for the former by amniocentesis is necessary, assessment of the mother's hepatitis B status is also important. Hepatitis B infection predisposes to hepatocellular carcinoma (increasing the risk by up to 200 times) and, if the fetus is normal, liver ultrasound scan, isotope study and possible CT scan should be performed to look for a space-occupying lesion.

Answer 16.10

The results are all normal and this boy has pseudopseudohypoparathyroidism. These patients have the physical stigmata of pseudohypoparathyroidism (the case quoted is typical) but normal biochemistry. Cataracts may develop despite a normal calcium concentration. Patients may have siblings with pseudohypoparathyroidism and can occasionally have raised parathyroid hormone levels.

Answer 17.1

There is an S wave in leads V1–V6 indicating clockwise rotation. The ST segment is depressed in leads V4–V6 and the T wave is asymmetrically inverted in the same leads. This is an ischaemic trace but without evidence of infarction.

Answer 17.2

This is a flat GTT curve and it is found in four groups of people:

- (*i*) Patients with malabsorption. However, a flat GTT is not by itself diagnostic of malabsorption.
- (*ii*) Patients with untreated Addison's disease—after replacement therapy the curve becomes normal.
- (*iii*) In people with growth hormone deficiency. The absence of growth hormone enhances muscle uptake of glucose.
- (*iv*) In otherwise normal people. This observation is unexplained.

Answer 17.3

(*a*) Porphyria cutanea tarda (PCT).
(*b*) Since his release from prison he had been living and sleeping in a local park. He had drunk large quantities of alcohol and had eaten little carbohydrate. The rash is photosensitive and over 90% of patients admit excess alcohol ingestion as the prelude to an acute attack. Chlorinated polycarbons have also been causal.

(c) Sunscreens may help the photodermatitis but he must abstain from alcohol. Venesection of one unit of blood a week until remission is achieved or the Hb falls below 12 g/dl is also helpful.

Answer 17.4

(a) Renal tubular acidosis Type IV.
(b) Hyporeninaemic hypoaldosteronism causes the hyperkalaemia, hyperchloraemia and acidosis seen here.
(c) Cyclosporin. Hyporeninaemic hypoaldosteronism is one of its side-effects and probably relates to renal tubular toxicity.
(d) Fludrocortisone corrects all of the biochemical abnormalities. The normal physiological replacement dose of 0.1–0.2 mg/day may be adequate but some patients may need as much as 0.6 mg/day. Patients may require sodium bicarbonate initially and they may also need a diuretic to compensate for the fluid-retaining effects of fludrocortisone. Cyclosporin dose reduction may correct the abnormality and the condition may be self limiting, even with continued treatment.

Answer 17.5

(a) The tracings are visual evoked potentials/responses (VEP/Rs). They are obtained by averaging-out the responses in the occipital leads of an electroencephalogram (EEG) to the repeated reversal of a chequerboard pattern of squares.
(b) They show a delay in the time of arrival of the response in the right eye. The response is also attenuated in amplitude and does not show the smaller negative components seen in the trace from the left eye. Demyelination or compression of the optic nerve can cause this. In this case they represent optic neuritis in a patient who has multiple sclerosis. Demyelinating plaques in the cervical spinal cord and ulnar nerve respectively account for the presenting symptoms and the occurrence of lesions at multiple sites is characteristic.

Answer 17.6

(a) This infant had Bartter's syndrome.
(b) A renal biopsy would show marked hypertrophy of the juxtaglomerular apparatus.

(c) The cause of the condition was considered to be a diminished ability of the proximal tubule to reabsorb sodium, leading to excess sodium reaching the distal tubule. The sodium and water loss reduces the extracellular fluid volume leading to a fall in blood pressure and raised renin, angiotensin and aldosterone. Subsequently it has been found that prostaglandin production (at least by the kidney) is much increased and if this is blocked by a drug such as indomethacin which inhibits prostaglandin synthetase virtually all parameters of the condition return to normal.

Answer 17.7

(a) The most likely diagnosis was rhesus incompatibility between fetus and mother.

(b) The differential diagnosis involved both rhesus and ABO incompatibilities.

(c) The further essential investigations were cord blood Coombs' test and the mother's blood and rhesus group. If the cord blood was Coombs' positive then the infant had rhesus incompatibility and the mother will be rhesus negative. From the given data the degree of rhesus incompatibility is mild as the haemoglobin is more than 12 g/dl and the bilirubin less than 68 μmol/l (4 mg/ 100 ml). If the cord blood was Coombs's negative then the diagnosis was an ABO incompatibility between mother and fetus. The maternal blood was very probably Group O because Group O incompatibility is much more common than any other blood group incompatibility.

Answer 17.8

(a) There are four skin diseases in which immunoglobulins and complement are deposited in uninvolved areas: pemphigus, pemphigoid, lupus erythematosus and dermatitis herpetiformis.

(b) In about 60% of patients with dermatitis herpetiformis the small bowel shows villous changes identical to those found in coeliac disease although patients are often asymptomatic.

(c) The intense pruritus of dermatitis herpetiformis responds within hours to oral dapsone and in time to a gluten-free diet in 70% of patients. Megaloblastic or haemolytic anaemia can be dangerous in elderly patients given dapsone.

Answer 17.9

(*a*) (*i*) Failure of the hypothalamic pituitary axis gonadotrophins such as occurs in pituitary tumours or hypogonadotrophic hypogonadism.
   (*ii*) Failure of gonadal response to gonadotrophins.
   (*iii*) Inability of sex steroid-dependent tissues to respond to normal output of sex hormones.
(*b*) The LH and FSH levels are in the postmenopausal range and the oestradiol level is low suggesting that the ovaries are failing to respond to gonadotrophins. The possible causes are gonadal agenesis; genotypic abnormalities (XO, Turner's; XY, testicular feminization); autoimmune ovarian failure, or ovarian destruction from radiotherapy or chemotherapy.

Answer 17.10

(*a*) Haemochromatosis.
(*b*) Cardiac dysfunction accounts for the dyspnoea and hypogonadism for the erectile failure and reduced beard growth. These are more common manifestations in this age group than the classic triad of liver disease, diabetes (which explains this man's polyuria) and skin pigmentation found in older patients.
(*c*) Venesection was the only treatment for some time but desferrioxamine by intravenous infusion or intramuscular injection is now known to be effective. Excessive venesection can produce cardiac failure and even death if there is severe iron-induced cardiac damage.

Answer 18.1

(*a*) This trace is an example of sinus bradycardia and sinus arrhythmia.
(*b*) Sinus bradycardia is a normal finding in young people and athletes. It is also found in association with digoxin treatment, β-blockade therapy, hypothermia, obstructive jaundice, hypothyroidism and raised intracranial pressure.

Answer 18.2

(*a*) The figures were those of an acute respiratory alkalosis (high pH but only slightly raised bicarbonate) and hypoxaemia.

(*b*) The differential diagnosis includes the following:

  (*i*) Multiple pulmonary emboli—risk factors are obesity, pelvic surgery and underlying malignancy (but ECG changes would be expected with this degree of hypoxia).

  (*ii*) Haemorrhage—an immediate haemoglobin may be misleading as there will have been no time for haemodilution.

  (*iii*) The early phase of 'shock lung' (adult respiratory distress syndrome—ARDS) prior to the development of hypercapnia and acidosis. Sepsis, disseminated intravascular coagulation (DIC) or fat embolism can cause ARDS.

Answer 18.3

There was a high bilirubin in the presence of a normal alkaline phosphatase and modestly elevated liver enzymes. The alkaline phosphatase concentration virtually excluded an obstructive lesion. The most likely diagnosis was postoperative jaundice associated with infection. Halothane hepatitis is also possible; minor hepatic dysfunction occurs in up to 20% of patients repeatedly exposed to it. Jaundice usually develops 1–3 weeks after exposure and severe hepatic necrosis occurs in 1 in 20–35 000 cases.

The differential diagnosis includes a previously unrecognized cirrhosis and an intrahepatic abscess.

Answer 18.4

(*a*) This patient had established acute renal failure. The U/P ratio for urea is 6.9 and for osmolarity is 1.08. Normally the U/P ratio for urea is 10 or more and the osmolarity U/P ratio is 2–3. If urea and osmolar ratios fall below 10 and 1.1 respectively, established acute renal failure is present. In addition in acute renal failure urine sodium is often more than 70 mmol/l (mEq/l).

(*b*) It is improbable that this patient would respond to intravenous fluid and an appropriate dose of a loop diuretic (frusemide or bumetanide). In a few patients there might be an increase in water excretion but no increase in concentrating ability of the kidney.

(c) An ultrasound scan should be performed to look for evidence of obstruction. A high-dose IVP may show a dense persistent nephrogram and give information about the renal size and shape. If it shows nothing on tomography then CT scanning after the contrast has been administered may be helpful.

Answer 18.5

These data show heart failure and motor neuropathy. Normally conduction velocity in the fastest fibres is about 60 m/s. Premature loss of hair pigmentation is associated with organ-specific autoimmune diseases. The differential diagnosis includes the following:

(i)   Diabetic heart failure due to ischaemic heart disease and neuropathy; the latter is usually predominantly sensory.
(ii) Amyloid disease.
(iii) Myxoedema.
(iv) Beriberi.

Answer 18.6

(a) The anion gap is calculated from the formula $(Na + K) - (Cl + HCO_3)$. Therefore $(145 + 5) - (98 + 20) = 32$.

(b) The gap represents approximately the sum of the unmeasured anions (protein, sulphate, phosphate, lactate and 3-hydroxybutyrate), the charges of which must, together with those of chloride and bicarbonate, balance those of the cations sodium and potassium. As charge is involved the constituents must be expressed in mEq/l and not mmol/l. The normal range is 12–17 mmol/l.

(c) The major causes of an increased gap are metabolic acidosis, severe renal failure, ketoacidosis, the acidotic phase of salicylate poisoning and lactic acidosis. Less common causes of metabolic acidosis include methanol and ethylene glycol (antifreeze) poisoning. In the presence of a normal blood glucose and plasma creatinine and the absence of salicylates, poisoning should be suspected and blood and urine sent to the local Poisons Centre.

It should be noted that a metabolic acidosis can occur in the presence of a normal anion gap. This is found when chloride has replaced bicarbonate as in renal tubular acidosis, ureterosigmoidostomy and in bicarbonate loss in severe persistent diarrhoea.

Answer 18.7

(a) This patient is likely to have pernicious anaemia. The high titre of antiparietal cell antibodies is suggestive of this diagnosis, and patients with ileal disease have an impaired ability to absorb vitamin B_{12} even in the presence of intrinsic factor—hence the negative Schilling test.

(b) Proof of pernicious anaemia in this patient could be obtained by measuring the reticulocyte count 5–8 days after the Schilling test (intramuscular vitamin B_{12}). A patient with pernicious anaemia responds maximally with a reticulocyte response of approximately 30% at this time.

Answer 18.8

(a) This woman experienced evening attacks of hypoglycaemia.
(b) This is a common feature in pregnant diabetics. Increased sensitivity to insulin occurs characteristically during the first trimester of pregnancy. The clinical picture may be confusing because glycosuria is not a feature of an ordinary hypoglycaemic episode. In this woman glycosuria represented the reduced renal threshold to glucose which is a normal feature of pregnancy.

Answer 18.9

(a) There is atrial fibrillation and complete AV block. Because of the block the atrial contractions are not conducted to the ventricles. The broad QRS complexes (rate 48/min) show a ventricular escape rhythm, perhaps suggesting that the block is below the AV node.
(b) A ventricular demand pacemaker is necessary because of the slow rate. The role of anticoagulants is controversial.

Answer 18.10

(*a*) This woman had taken Co-proxamol tablets; they contain dextropropoxyphene hydrochloride 32.5 mg and paracetamol (acetaminophen) 325 mg in each tablet. The paracetamol component explains the liver and renal dysfunction.

(*b*) Naloxone: dextropropoxyphene is an opiate derivative and its central nervous system effects can be reversed by narcotic antagonists.

Answer 19.1

(*a*) (*i*) There is an RSR′ pattern in leads V4–V6, the S waves in leads V1–V3 are deep slurred and in V4–V6 notched with ST depression; and there is T wave inversion in leads V4–V6.

(*ii*) The S wave in V1 plus the R wave in V5 is 40 mm.

(*b*) The features described in (*i*) are indicative of left bundle branch block. The trace is always pathological and may be found in ischaemic heart disease, hypertension, aortic valvular disease and following cardiac surgery. Left ventricular hypertrophy is indicated by (*ii*). There is some debate whether voltage criteria for LVH hold in all cases when LBBB is present.

Answer 19.2

(*a*) The association of healed rib fractures and extensive mottling of the lungs is virtually diagnostic of skid-row tuberculosis. Fractures occur in brawls or when drunk or both.

(*b*) Sputum or gastric aspirate would yield *Mycobacterium tuberculosis*. Anaemia—iron deficient or macrocytic—is common. Obstructive lung disease may be detected by blood gas measurments or spirometry. Liver function tests may suggest alcoholic hepatitis or cirrhosis although miliary TB should also be considered.

Answer 19.3

(*a*) This man had polycythaemia rubra vera. The sudden abdominal symptoms with mild jaundice and raised liver enzymes are suggestive of a development of hepatic venous obstruction

(Budd–Chiari syndrome). One would expect enlargement of the liver and ascites to develop.

(b) The Budd–Chiari syndrome is an occasional complication of polycythaemia rubra vera but in many cases the aetiology is unexplained.

(c) The generally poor uptake of isotope by the liver is to be expected; in some people the caudate lobe may have venous drainage to the infradiaphragmatic portion of the inferior vena cava other than by one of the main hepatic veins. It may therefore be spared during a thrombotic episode and excess isotope will accumulate in this region.

(d) An inferior vena cavagram is indicated to demonstrate a characteristic narrowing distortion of the vein throughout its intrahepatic course.

Answer 19.4

(a) This man had primary hyperaldosteronism (Conn's syndrome). There was hypertension with low renin and a high plasma aldosterone. The normal response to a low sodium diet is an increase in renin concentration but in the presence of an adrenal adenoma producing aldosterone the response is blocked.

(b) CT scanning may localize the tumour to one adrenal gland but measurement of renal venous aldosterone may be necessary before deciding on which side to operate.

(c) Definitive treatment is surgical removal of the adenoma after which there is a good chance that the blood pressure will return to normal and remain so. The condition may be treated with spironolactone which is very effective but expensive and its side-effects (gynaecomastia, hirsuties and gastric intolerance) may be limiting in some patients.

Answer 19.5

(a) These findings are typical of Froin's syndrome. Apart from a much-raised protein content the CSF pressure failed to vary with the respiration or jugular compression (Queckenstedt's test). The commonest cause of this syndrome is an advanced spinal tumour or an area of spinal meningitis.

(b) The differential diagnosis is that of raised CSF protein which at this high concentration includes the Guillain–Barré syndrome and some intracranial tumours especially an acoustic neuroma. The CSF protein is very high at the onset of symptoms in spinal block due to tumour of the cord, whereas in Guillain–Barré syndrome it may be only a little raised at the onset but continues to rise even though the symptoms begin to remit.

Answer 19.6

The most likely diagnosis is eclampsia. The explanation is as follows: proteinuria of 3–4 g/day is insufficient to cause hypo-albuminaemic oedema. The serum urate is raised in eclampsia and is disproportionately high for a creatinine clearance of 78 ml/min due to primary renal causes. Hypertension, oedema and convulsions are the triad that comprises eclampsia and lactosuria can be found in pregnant women.

Answer 19.7

(a) This man had sideroblastic anaemia. The features are a fairly severe anaemia with dimorphic red blood cells with a raised serum iron and normal or raised iron-binding capacity.
(b) The marrow would show an increase in iron stores—a greater number and size of iron granules. In some marrow cells the iron granules form a peripheral ring in the cytoplasm: sideroblasts.
(c) It may be a primary hereditary condition, secondary to drugs (e.g. alcohol or chloramphenicol) or toxins (e.g. lead), associated with myeloproliferative disease (e.g. chronic myeloid leukaemia or polycythaemia rubra vera), haemolytic anaemia or collagen vascular diseases.

Answer 19.8

These results may be obtained in relation to pregnancy, the use of oral contraceptives or oestrogen therapy. In each of these circumstances there is an increase in thyroid-binding globulin and there is thus an increased quantity of bound thyroxine raising the serum concentration despite a euthyroid status.

Answer 19.9

(a) This woman had nephrotic syndrome: oedema, hypo-albuminaemia and proteinuria of more than 5 g daily.

(b) With a background of non-organ specific autoimmune disease it is possible that a similar disease process had developed—systemic lupus erythematosus with renal involvement. Alternatively renal amyloid, an occasional complication of Still's disease, may have developed. Renal damage secondary to long-continued analgesics should be considered but is excluded by the normal IVP. The nephrotic syndrome may be secondary to gold or penicillamine therapy when the renal biopsy is likely to show membranous glomerulonephritis.

(c) The antinuclear factor (ANF) should be measured and a renal biopsy undertaken. In this woman the ANF was not present and many glomeruli contained amyloid deposits. Some patients with renal amyloid excrete λ and $\varkappa$ light chains in the urine. The explanation is not clear but it is thought that during a long-continued inflammatory process excess immunoglobulin (antibody) is formed, some of the light chains of which are excreted in the urine.

Answer 19.10

(a) This patient had anticonvulsant osteomalacia.

(b) The condition is quite widely recognized in patients who need to take long-term anticonvulsants in large doses, in particular phenytoin and phenobarbitone.

(c) It is thought that non-specific hepatic induction by the anticonvulsant impairs vitamin D_3 hydroxylation with an increase in more polar inactive metabolites. There was therefore less 25-OHD$_3$ to be further hydroxylated to 1,25-(OH)$_2$D$_3$, the active derivative responsible for maintaining calcium homeostasis. There may also be increased degradation of 1,25-(OH)$_2$D$_3$ to inactive metabolites.

In chronic biliary cirrhosis similar vitamin D metabolic abnormalities may develop and osteomalacia may occur.

Answer 20.1

(a) This rhythm strip shows a second-degree heart block (Wenckebach type).

(b) The ST elevation indicates a recent infarction but its site and extent cannot be stated from a rhythm strip alone.

Answer 20.2

The patient had a rheumatoid effusion. Such an effusion is differentiated from an effusion complicating systemic lupus erythematosus (SLE), as shown in the *Table:*

	Rheumatoid arthritis	*SLE*
pH	<7.2	>7.35
Glucose concentration	<1.4 mmol/l (<25 mg/100 ml)	4.4 mmol/l (80 mg/100 ml) or more
LDH	>700 iu/l	500 iu/l or less

In addition, rheumatoid effusions contain antinuclear antibodies, IgM rheumatoid factor, ragocytes, (macrophages with IgM-containing inclusions) and immune complexes at higher concentrations than in the circulation.

Answer 20.3

(a) This woman had primary biliary cirrhosis despite the presence of hypercupriuria, hypercupraemia and a raised liver copper concentration. The raised copper concentrations are suggestive of Wilson's disease but the normal concentration of ceruloplasmin is much against this diagnosis. Some compounds accumulate in the plasma in severe liver disease and result in an artefactually low ceruloplasmin concentration. The result may also be low due to reduced protein synthesis which occurs in severe liver failure. The mild jaundice and mild elevation of alanine transaminase with a very raised alkaline phosphatase in a middle-aged woman is very suggestive of primary biliary cirrhosis.

(b) This would be confirmed by finding a high titre of antimicrosomal antibodies. This antibody is present in the serum of about 95% of patients with primary biliary cirrhosis.

Answer 20.4

(a) This man had many features of a generalized proximal renal tubular defect. There was a tubular type of proteinuria, generalized amino-aciduria and raised phosphate clearance (implied by the subnormal plasma concentration), impaired ability to acidify the urine, reduced urinary concentrating power and a border-line systemic acidosis. All these features are compatible with the adult Fanconi syndrome and associated renal tubular acidosis type II.

(b) The glycosuria is of the renal type and a standard glucose tolerance test would have a normal or 'flat' curve.

Answer 20.5

(a) This is a macular cortical lesion.

(b) It is caused by damage to the tip of the occipital pole.

(c) Direct trauma, head injury or bullet wounds produce these homonymous macular defects. These may be incomplete but are always exactly congruous.

Answer 20.6

(a) This boy was exhibiting the rare Lesch–Nyhan syndrome. The combination of the neurological features and the excessively raised serum urate makes the diagnosis. The macrocytic anaemia is not due to folate deficiency but may respond to adenine supplements.

(b) The disease is a sex-linked recessive inborn error of metabolism in which there is a lack of the enzyme hypoxanthine-guanine phosphoribosyl transferase (HGPRT). This enzyme catalyses the conversion of hypoxanthine and guanine to their respective nucleotides—inosinic acid and guanylic acid. In the absence of HGPRT an excess of hypoxanthine and xanthine develops which is metabolized to urate by xanthine oxidase. It is thought that the features of the Lesch–Nyhan syndrome result from accumulation of purine metabolites (hypoxanthine and guanine) in neuronal cells (particularly the basal ganglia). In other areas of the brain (putamen and caudate nucleus) a decrease in dopa decarboxylase and tyrosine hydroxylase has also been found.

Answer 20.7

(a) The ECG is that of pulmonary hypertension. There is right axis deviation with a dominant S in lead I together with enlarged P waves (P pulmonale) and dominant R waves in the right chest leads.

(b) This may therefore be the ECG of cor pulmonale secondary to chronic bronchitis with a secondary polycythaemia. The ECG would also fit a pulmonary embolic or thrombolic episode which is a complication of primary polycythaemia.

Answer 20.8

(a) The symptoms and high urinary catecholamine levels suggest either a phaeochromocytoma or the rebound phenomenon which occurs in some patients who withdraw their regular doses of clonidine abruptly.

(b) This man had left his supply of clonidine at home. The explanation of this phenomenon is not known but it is believed that during clonidine treatment there is increased storage of catecholamine in nerve terminals by the stimulation of inhibitory α-receptors. If the drug is suddenly stopped the stored amines are released, mimicking phaeochromocytomata both clinically and biochemically.

(c) In the acute phase the treatment of choice is clonidine—symptoms subside rapidly and blood pressure is lowered. Alternatively labetalol may be used which has α- and β-blocking properties and can also be given parenterally.

Answer 20.9

(a) The history is typical of polymyalgia rheumatica in which there was giant cell arteritis of the right temporal and ophthalmic arteries. From 30% to 50% of patients presenting with temporal arteritis have evidence of polymyalgia rheumatica when a detailed history is taken and examination performed.

(b) The diagnosis is established by a biopsy of the tender superficial temporal artery (or other involved artery of the scalp or occiput).

(c) The condition is treated with prednisolone 40–60 mg daily.

(d) Treatment must be begun at once before the histological diagnosis is made. Biopsies performed within 24 h of starting steroid treatment still show characteristic histological changes. If treatment is delayed, thrombotic occlusion of the involved arteries occurs which in this patient would have led to blindness of the right eye and necrosis of the area supplied by the superficial temporal artery. High-dose prednisolone is continued until the ESR is normal and then very slowly reduced as the condition may relapse acutely.

Answer 20.10

(a) A thiazide diuretic. There is typically a reduced urate and calcium excretion and also an increase in urinary magnesium and iodide excretion.

(b) Acute gout is occasionally precipitated by thiazides due to retention of urate. Thiazides also have a diabetogenic effect.

(c) The ability to reduce calcium excretion with thiazide diuretics is of value in idiopathic hypercalcuria. Urine calcium may fall by as much as one-third with bendrofluazide and this property is used to augment other measures in reducing calcium excretion and hence stone formation in these patients.

Answer 21.1

(a) This rhythm strip shows atrial fibrillation with ventricular extrasystoles. There is an R on T phenomenon and the final portion of the strip shows ventricular fibrillation.

(b) Treatment includes: closed chest massage; intubation and 100% oxygen administration; setting up a drip; intravenous lignocaine; intravenous bicarbonate; DC shock.

Answer 21.2

(a) He now has type II respiratory failure (ventilatory failure).

(b) He had been given oxygen at too high a concentration. This is shown by the greatly raised P_{CO_2} of 141 mmHg (18.8 kPa) and the P_{O_2} of 108 mmHg (14.4 kPa). Patients with chronic obstructive airways disease lose the usual stimulatory effect of hypercapnia on the respiratory centre as the P_{CO_2} is chronically raised. Their respiratory drive relies on the hypoxic stimulus and if this is removed because the inspired oxygen tension (P_{IO_2}) is raised by supplementary oxygen then ventilatory failure occurs. Respiratory failure is defined as $Pco_2 > 55\,mmHg$ ($7.3\,kPa$) and/or $Po_2 < 45\,mmHg$ ($6.0\,kPa$).

(c) Apart from chest deformities associated with longstanding bronchitis, this man was semiconscious, not coughing, not cyanosed and had papilloedema.

(d) Further treatment is urgent and ideally involves transfer to an intensive care unit. Inspired oxygen in a concentration of 24% should be given. Intubation and aspiration of lung secretions may also be needed. Bronchodilators should be given via nebulizer (both β agonists and anticholinergics) and steroids intravenously. The role of the respiratory stimulant doxapram is controversial.

Answer 21.3

The data presented here are compatible with Gilbert's hyperbilirubinaemia in which the only abnormality is a mild elevation of total bilirubin.

(a) Mild hyperbilirubinaemia in the absence of any abnormality of hepatic cellular function, haemolytic jaundice or obstruction to bile drainage suggests a familial or constitutional hyperbilirubinaemia. In the Dubin–Johnson type, hyperbilirubinaemia may be much greater and the liver biopsy shows normal architecture with an excess of an abnormal pigment which resembles melanin. The Rotor type of hyperbilirubinaemia is biochemically very similar to the Dubin–Johnson but the liver biopsy is not pigmented. The Crigler–Najjar hyperbilirubinaemia presents in childhood and a diagnosis would not have been delayed to the age of 40 years as in this case. The very rare primary shunt hyperbilirubinaemia is associated with very high levels of urinary urobilinogen and reticulocytosis may be present.

(b) A liver biopsy is not indicated.

(c) If patients with Gilbert's disease are fasted for 36–48 hours plasma bilirubin tends to rise further, which gives some confirmation of the diagnosis in this condition which is entirely benign.

Answer 21.4

(a) This woman had a postabortion haemolytic anaemia with haemoglobinaemia and bilirubinaemia (black/red urine). The high white blood cell count reflected both the haemolytic anaemia and the presence of infection—most probably due to *Clostridium welchii* as this organism is frequently recovered in patients with septic abortion. *Clostridium welchii* produces a lecithinase which disrupts red blood cells and platelets.

(*b*) Complications include: (*i*) septicaemia; (*ii*) disseminated intravascular coagulation (possibly already present; see platelet count); (*iii*) acute renal failure; (*iv*) cortical necrosis; (*v*) death.

Answer 21.5

(*a*) This is likely to result from an embolus in a branch of the central retinal artery. The central retinal artery divides into upper and lower branches which supply the retina above and below the horizontal meridian of the eye. Occlusion of a branch causes a defect that extends only to the horizontal meridian.

(*b*) The commonest causes of retinal artery occlusion are cholesterol crystals from an atheromatous plaque in a large artery, emboli composed of fibrin or platelets, or fragments from an aortic valve (either calcified or affected by endocarditis).

Answer 21.6

This patient had all the clinical features of Marfan's syndrome. In those patients in whom dislocation of the lens occurs it is important to test for homocystinuria (cystathionine synthetase deficiency) as many patients with homocystinuria have the same body configuration as in Marfan's syndrome.

Answer 21.7

The second portion of the Schilling test would have to be performed—oral labelled vitamin B_{12} together with oral intrinsic factor. Eleven per cent recovery is in the low normal range for most patients without vitamin B_{12} deficiency anaemia. If the amount of radioactivity in the urine then increased this would be diagnostic of intrinsic factor deficiency and hence pernicious anaemia.

Answer 21.8

(a) Lithium. Hypothyroidism with hypercalcaemia are recognized complications of lithium therapy.
(b) Also described are: nephrogenic diabetes insipidus, possible exacerbation of psoriasis, mania, reversible T-wave flattening and interaction with haloperidol leading to prolonged extrapyramidal symptoms.

Answer 21.9

(a) The overnight urine osmolarity is low; in the absence of renal disease, figures above 700 mmol/l are usual.
(b) This man had mild diabetes insipidus. It is now well recognized that lithium has an effect on water metabolism. Thirst occurs in 40% of patients taking lithium but only 10–15% develop nephrogenic diabetes insipidus.

Answer 21.10

He has Gaisbock's syndrome or relative ('stress') polycythaemia and probable excessive alcohol intake. The PCV is raised but he has a normal red blood cell volume—and therefore a reduced plasma volume. The transaminases are raised and the ferritin and serum B_{12} are approaching the upper limit of normal while the red cell folate approaches the lower limit of normal in the presence of a slightly high MCV. These features all occur in the setting of excessive consumption of alcohol which is a common cause of relative polycythaemia. Smoking, which often accompanies this, contributes to polycythaemia by a reduction in plasma volume and may increase the red cell volume.

Answer 22.1

(a) These chest leads show a complete right bundle branch block.
(b) There is an RSR' pattern in leads V1–V3 and wide slurred S waves in leads V5 and V6.

(c) Right bundle branch block may be found in: normal people; pulmonary embolism; chronic lung disease leading to right ventricular hypertrophy; congenital heart disease such as ASD; ischaemic heart disease; hypertensive heart disease; rheumatic heart disease; post cardiac surgery.

Answer 22.2

(a) It is generally agreed that patients with primary gout have an increased incidence of Type IV hyperlipoproteinaemia.

(b) This condition usually presents with abdominal pain due to pancreatitis or crops of eruptive xanthomata on the extensor surfaces of the arms and legs. There is also a link with impaired glucose tolerance and diabetes.

(c) The plasma in Type IV hyperlipoproteinaemia is turbid due to a raised triglyceride concentration of about 2–10 mmol/l (175–885 mg/100 ml) and at times with cholesterol elevation (type V hyperlipoproteinaemia). There is an increase in the pre-β-lipoproteins with very high very-low-density lipoprotein (VLDL) concentrations and low levels of low- and high-density lipoprotein (LDL and HDL). There is reduced synthesis of apoprotein A-I (Apo A-I) and the condition is autosomal dominant.

Answer 22.3

(a) This woman had hypophosphataemia, hyperglycaemia and hypokalaemic alkalosis. The symptoms and biochemical findings may occur in patients who are being fed intravenously, especially those who are already nutritionally depleted.

(b) The symptoms are due to the hypophosphataemia which is more marked if additional insulin is given. Hypophosphataemia is very probably due to the rapid acceleration of glucose phosphory-lation induced by dextrose infusion with consequent cellular uptake of inorganic phosphorus from the plasma. The hypoka-laemic alkalosis is a reflection upon rapid cellular uptake of circulating potassium.

(c) In parenteral nutrition, concentrated sugar solutions are essential for energy requirements and are usually combined with lipid emulsions and amino acid mixtures. Phosphate, additional to that available in intravenous lipid preparations, should be given so that the patient receives about 0.5–0.7 mmol (1.5–2.2 mg/dl) phosphate/kg bodyweight daily, provided that renal function is normal.

Answer 22.4

The diagnosis was compulsive water drinking. The differential diagnosis is between pituitary diabetes insipidus and compulsive water drinking. In compulsive water drinking the plasma osmolarity tends to be less than 290 mmol/l and in diabetes insipidus above 290 mmol/l. If a patient with pituitary diabetes insipidus is treated with vasopressin the polyuria and thirst cease and the urine osmolarity rises. In patients with compulsive water drinking, vasopressin has a much less marked effect as their thirst is not related to polyuria but to their neurotic personalities. Water intoxication may develop in this circumstance.

Answer 22.5

(a) E—the dorsal columns.
(b) The sensory modalities of proprioception, vibration and deep pain are carried in the dorsal columns. The spinothalamic tracts (A and B) carry touch sensation.
(c) Syphilis causes tabes dorsalis by damaging these pathways selectively. Vitamin B_{12} deficiency and Friedreich's ataxia must also be considered in the differential diagnosis.

Answer 22.6

(a) Severe backache and abnormalities of micturition in an elderly man suggest carcinoma of the prostate with metastases to vertebrae. In this patient the acid phosphatase was raised, as is the rule with secondary forms of this neoplasm. The raised alkaline phosphatase reflected bone osteoblastic activity around the site of the metastases.
(b) The bone origin of the alkaline phosphatase could be confirmed by electrophoresis of the enzyme. The prostatic carcinoma should be confirmed by prostatic biopsy and the vertebral disease by X-ray and radioisotope bone scan, which will show sclerotic areas and 'hot spots' respectively, corresponding to the metastases.

Answer 22.7

(a) 102–110 fl (μm^3) because there is vitamin B_{12} deficiency and also iron deficiency so the MCV is not as high as would be seen in pure vitamin B_{12} deficiency.

(b) There will be depressed absorption of vitamin B_{12} with and without intrinsic factor.

(c) The bacteria which overgrow in the stagnant loop of bowel may synthesize folate which is absorbed and leads to supranormal serum concentrations.

(d) The upper small gut is normally sterile; a blind loop becomes colonized by large numbers of coliform and bacteroides species. The organisms compete for available vitamin B_{12} and may consume sufficient to produce a megaloblastic anaemia. Malabsorption of iron also occurs as well as that of fats because of splitting of bile salts by the blind loop bacteria into compounds which are toxic to the mucosa of the small gut.

Answer 22.8

No precise diagnosis can be made from the data given. She probably does not have Conn's syndrome (primary hyperaldosteronism) because:

(i) the plasma aldosterone was in the normal range;

(ii) while she was mildly hypokalaemic there was no accompanying alkalosis which is almost invariable in Conn's syndrome;

(iii) spironolactone will reduce the blood pressure to normal in patients other than those who have Conn's syndrome.

Answer 22.9

This patient had a macrocytic anaemia and steatorrhoea. This anaemia commonly accompanies chronic liver disease and perhaps reflects hepatic inability to store vitamin B_{12}. Steatorrhoea occurred following the increased neomycin dosage. Neomycin causes steatorrhoea and malabsorption by two mechanisms: it produces reversible and modest gut mucosal damage and also combines with bile and fatty acids leading to disruption of micelles.

Answer 22.10

(*a*) (*i*) Excessive water intake: hysterical polydipsia or a relative excess of dextrose in the intravenous regimen.

(*ii*) Excessive water retention: syndrome of inappropriate ADH secretion (SIADH).

(*iii*) Excessive sodium loss: either from the gastrointestinal tract (vomiting or diarrhoea) or the kidneys (usually tubulo-interstitial disease or hypoadrenalism—Addison's syndrome).

(*b*) The diagnosis was Addison's disease; although not hyperkalaemic she is mildly acidotic. In SIADH urinary sodium is approximately 50 mmol/l and in sodium depletion due to excessive loss urinary sodium is very low (< 20 mmol/l).

Answer 23.1

(*a*) and (*b*) The ST segment is elevated concave upwards in leads V2–V6. These are the classic findings of acute pericarditis. The ST elevation of an acute infarction is concave downwards.

(*c*) The patient is likely to have had central chest pain similar to that experienced with ischaemic heart disease. Pericardial pain tends to show postural variation while that of ischaemic heart disease does not.

Answer 23.2

(*a*) The first point to notice is the systemic alkalosis associated with a raised urea. If this urea were a reflection of renal parenchymal damage the bicarbonate would be in the normal range. The next step is to calculate the plasma chloride: $(Na + K) - (HCO_3 + Cl)$ = anion gap. Therefore $Cl = 138 - 44 = 94$. This patient was therefore depleted of sodium, chloride and potassium. These features together with the alkalosis are typical of persistent vomiting due to pyloric stenosis.

(*b*) Sodium and potassium are lost in the vomitus but proportionately more hydrogen and chloride ions are lost. Gastric juice contains approximately sodium 50, chloride 45, potassium 12 and hydrogen 50 mmol/l. The renal response to persistent vomiting is to conserve sodium at the expense of potassium and hydrogen ions. Because of the loss of hydrogen ions from the stomach, alkalosis develops and this effect is additive to the renal exchange of potassium and hydrogen ions for sodium ions. The urine is likely to be acid (pH < 7) despite the systemic alkalosis.

Answer 23.3

Raised IgM and positive antimitochondrial antibodies strongly suggest a diagnosis of primary biliary cirrhosis. They are also found in chronic active hepatitis but this condition is rarely associated with a neutral or alkaline pH (renal tubular acidosis) when there is a 60% association between primary biliary cirrhosis and renal tubular acidosis. Haematemesis secondary to oesophageal varices may occur in patients with primary biliary cirrhosis and there is an increased incidence of peptic ulceration.

Answer 23.4

(a) This man had osteomalacia and nephrocalcinosis. These two findings alone are very suggestive of adult (distal) renal tubular acidosis (RTA) type I. There was no evidence of malabsorption from the gut in this patient and he had a neutral to only mildly acidic urine in the presence of a systemic acidosis—compatible with RTA.

(b) The definitive investigation is the demonstration of failure of the urine pH to fall below 5.4 after an acid load—usually given as ammonium chloride 0.1 g/kg bodyweight. In RTA type I there is an inability to maintain a gradient of hydrogen ions across the distal renal tubule: a persistent acidosis results which impairs maintenance of bone calcification with resulting osteomalacia.

Answer 23.5

(a) A and B—the anterior and lateral spinothalamic (cortico-spinal) tracts respectively.

(b) These tracts carry pain and temperature sensation. The majority of the fibres decussate immediately after entering the cord but a few (in Lissauer's tract) spread upwards and downwards on the same side for two or three segments before decussating.

(c) The sensory level is approximately T9 and there is a partial Brown-Séquard syndrome. Extrinsic unilateral spinal cord compression by a dorsal root neurofibroma, meningioma or dural metastatic deposit could cause this, as could TB or a pyogenic extradural abscess.

Answer 23.6

(a) (i) Hypernatraemia secondary to gastroenteritis; (ii) renal insufficiency precipitated by infection on the basis of congenitally abnormal kidneys; (iii) adrenogenital syndrome; (iv) transient neonatal hyperglycaemia; (v) nephrogenic diabetes insipidus.

(b) Additional investigations include urine sample for microscopy and culture, stool culture, blood culture, blood glucose measurement, urine collection for assay of 17-ketosteroids, 17-hydroxycorticosteroids, and IVP.

The probable cause is infection of the gastrointestinal tract. Diarrhoea may be a non-specific symptom and the infection should be looked for in other areas—urine and blood particularly. If the infection is in the urinary tract an underlying congenital abnormality of the renal tract should be subsequently excluded.

If the dehydration appears disproportionate to the preceding symptoms, underlying metabolic disorders should be considered (e.g. adrenogenital syndrome). Urinary pregnanediol, gonadotrophins and 17-ketosteroids are elevated.

Gross elevation of blood glucose with hyperosmolar dehydration is found in transient neonatal diabetes mellitus—which is rare.

Answer 23.7

(a) Assuming that this patient had vitamin B_{12} deficiency due to pernicious anaemia, the most common explanation of failure of treatment is the co-existence of an iron deficiency anaemia.

(b) A megaloblastic marrow could be due to vitamin B_{12} deficiency but there may be a co-existence of folate deficiency, which may be dietary in origin or related to pregnancy or cirrhosis. Folate malabsorption may occur in bowel diseases or may be related to an anticonvulsant, folic acid antagonist (methotrexate) or use of the oral contraceptive.

Hence megaloblastic anaemias should be fully investigated before any treatment is given.

Answer 23.8

(*a*) This child exhibited the Di George syndrome. This consists of aplasia of the thymus and parathyroid deficiency, presumably due to malformation of the third and fourth branchial pouches. Lymphocytes which form spontaneous rosettes with sheep red blood cells are T-cells—lymphocytes which have been processed by the thymus to become immunologically competent and are then able to aid in defence against infection.

(*b*) Lymph node biopsy will show the bursa-dependent zones to be normally populated but the thymus-dependent zones (paracortical areas) will contain no lymphocytes.

(*c*) A fetal thymus graft surgically implanted into the rectus sheath will restore the immune system to normal in the Di George syndrome.

Answer 23.9

(*a*) She has polycystic ovary disease and shows a typically raised LH and low normal FSH. The testosterone concentration is raised resulting in hirsutism which is a common presenting complaint. Prolactinomas can cause infertility but they give rise to high prolactin concentrations (usually >1000 iU/l). Congenital adrenal hyperplasia can present in this manner but would give rise to a raised urinary ketosteroid excretion.

(*b*) Ultrasound is usually diagnostic of the condition but occasionally laparoscopy is required.

(*c*) Endometrial carcinoma is more common in these patients, presumably due to the prolonged oestrogen effects unopposed by luteal phase progesterones.

Answer 23.10

(*a*) Phenytoin may cause a macrocytic anaemia and low white blood cell count. Induction of liver enzymes causes increased metabolism of vitamin D to inactive products and therefore osteomalacia—manifest by the raised alkaline phosphatase and low urinary calcium excretion.

(*b*) Phenytoin may cause lymphadenopathy, gum hypertrophy, hirsutism, coarse facies, Dupytren's contracture, peripheral neuropathy and a rash.

(c) Alcohol can induce liver enzymes and result in a very similar picture and although he is unlikely to have consumed enough by this age it is not impossible.

Answer 24.1

(a) The strip shows ventricular bigeminy. Apart from the ventricular beats the other complexes are normal.

(b) This ECG finding may be found in: apparently normal people; ischaemic heart disease; digoxin toxicity; cardiomyopathies.

Answer 24.2

A: Normal

B: Uncompensated respiratory alkalosis as in acute hyperventilation which may be either psychogenic or reflex in response to acute pulmonary pathology (e.g. pulmonary embolism).

C: Uncompensated respiratory acidosis as in acute and chronic chest diseases including severe asthma, stridor and flail chests.

D: Compensated respiratory acidosis—the pH has been returned to normal by a metabolic alkalosis. This occurs in gross obesity, ankylosing spondylitis, poliomyelitis.

E: Uncompensated metabolic acidosis as seen in aspirin overdose, diabetic ketoacidosis, advanced renal failure and lactic acidosis. Given a steady rate of hydrogen ion production leading to a metabolic acidosis and subsequent renal compensation, arterial pH will rise to 7.35–7.4 but the plasma bicarbonate will remain at about 12–15 mmol/l (mEq/l).

Answer 24.3

(a) The woman had tetany and inflammatory bowel disease.

(b) Serum magnesium—it was 0.49 mmol/l (0.98 mEq/l).

(c) Patients with severe and prolonged diarrhoea may develop hypomagnesaemia. Very rarely is malabsorption a cause.

Answer 24.4

These figures are compatible with:

(*i*) Pregnancy: the GFR and hence the creatinine clearance rises to 40–50% above normal from about the third to eighth month of pregnancy and glycosuria is found in up to 40% of pregnant women as the Tm_G falls.

(*ii*) Nephrotic syndrome: raised creatinine clearance is found in some of these patients due to an increased renal loss of creatinine. In addition, glycosuria is found in some nephrotic patients due to tubular dysfunction.

(*iii*) Acromegaly: the GFR and hence the creatinine clearance rises due to increased renal size secondary to growth hormone. In addition, diabetes is common in acromegalics.

Answer 24.5

(*a*) C—the central canal.

(*b*) The fibres carrying pain and temperature sensation which decussate almost immediately after entering the cord are damaged as they cross the midline. As the lesion spreads laterally the reflex arcs are blocked and the pyramidal tract (F) may be damaged.

(*c*) The level is approximately T1. Syringomyelia, glioma, astrocytoma or ependymoma are possible causes.

(*d*) A right-sided Horner's syndrome may occur as the sympathetic fibres travelling in the motor root of T1 to synapse in Clarke's column are compressed.

Answer 24.6

(*a*) There was a hypokalaemic alkalosis in the presence of normal renal function.

(*b*) (*i*) Long-term diuretic therapy; this is the commonest cause.

(*ii*) Corticosteroid therapy; the sodium-retaining (mineralocorticoid) properties of the steroid causes secondary renal potassium loss.

(*iii*) Cushing's disease: the same mechanism operates as in (*ii*).

(*iv*) Conn's syndrome: aldosterone excess causes sodium retention and potassium loss.

(*v*) Excess dosage of carbenoxolone sodium in the treatment of gastric ulcer. Carbenoxolone has a renal potassium excretory effect as has liquorice, which is also used in the treatment of ulcer and can be obtained as confectionery which, if taken in excess, can produce the same picture.

(*vi*) Purgative abuse. Potassium is the major ion of the large bowel; excess purgation leads to potassium depletion.

Answer 24.7

(*a*) There was anaemia, thrombocytopenia and abnormalities of clotting. The rubella HAI titre was normal. Possibly his 'German measles' was some other viral infection since the clinical diagnosis is inexact.

(*b*) Acute promyelocytic leukaemia, with evidence of disseminated intravascular coagulation (DIC). The latter is a common feature in this leukaemia.

(*c*) A blood film will contain blast cells although a careful search may be needed. A bone marrow aspirate will consist mainly of blast cells.

(*d*) Treatment is less successful than for acute lymphoblastic leukaemia. Combinations of daunorubicin, cytosine arabinoside (ara-c) and 6-thioguanine (DAT) are the most successful.

Answer 24.8

(*a*) The albumin and α_1-globulin peaks are reduced and there is an obvious increase in the gamma region with fusion of the beta and gamma regions (compare with normal, *Figure 31.3*).

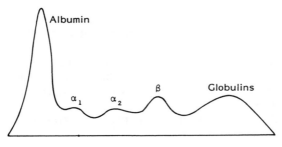

Figure 31.3

(*b*) Assuming the electrophoresis was of serum the most likely diagnosis is cirrhosis, in which all the above features are found. The other possible diagnosis is nephrotic syndrome, but in this condition α_1-globulin is very frequently increased in concentration and the gamma globulin concentration is less frequently raised than in cirrhosis.

If the electrophoresis was of urine, the patient would have had a proteinuria of more than 15 g daily and this would have been of the non-selective type.

Answer 24.9

(*a*) Blood sugar and arterial blood gases. The blood glucose was 54 mmol/l and she had a severe metabolic acidosis with a pH of 6.85.

(*b*) She was a newly diagnosed diabetic presenting with keto-acidosis (DKA). Low plasma sodium concentrations occur in DKA because of movement of intracellular water into the extracellular compartment. This is compounded by an osmotic diuresis in which a relative excess of salt may be lost. Vomiting and replacement of losses by drinking water may also dilute the extracellular space.

(*c*) This result is artefactually low due to hypertriglyceridaemia which makes interpretation impossible. However, the expected normal plasma sodium concentration should be reduced by 1 mmol/l for every 6 mmol/l of glucose present when assessing the degree of sodium depletion. In this case a plasma sodium of 140 − (54/6) = 131 mmol/l would be considered to be normal.

Answer 24.10

(*a*) Coeliac disease

(*b*) There is malabsorption of folate, vitamin B_{12}, iron, vitamin D and calcium.

(*c*) HLA B8 occurs in 80% of patients with coeliac disease compared with 20% of the general population.

(*d*) Wheat, barley, rye (and probably oats) contain gluten and should be avoided. This should relieve symptoms and improve nutrition and, according to some evidence, reduce the risk of lymphoma.

Answer 25.1

(*a*) This ECG strip shows a supraventricular tachycardia with bundle branch block. There is a rapid sequence of regular complexes (rate 165) and the QRS is widened, which is not infrequent during rapid supraventricular rhythms resulting from either aberrant conduction or bundle branch block. The last three QRS complexes show a sinus tachycardia.

(*b*) Attacks may often be aborted by manoeuvres to increase vagal tone such as carotid sinus massage, pressure on the globe of the eye or by the Valsalva manoeuvre (NB: vagal tone increases after stopping forced expiration, not during it).

(*c*) Resistant cases may respond to digoxin or practolol alone or combined. Verapamil may be used but if so should not be used with β-blockers. Cardioversion may be required.

Answer 25.2

(*a*) She is vitamin D deficient, due either to severe malabsorption or to dietary deficiency, and would probably manifest clinical signs of rickets. The phosphate would be elevated if she had chronic renal failure.

(*b*) Symptoms will be of bone pain—clinical bone deformity may be demonstrable. There may also be a proximal myopathy which can be severe enough to lead to confinement to a wheelchair or may merely make climbing stairs very difficult.

Answer 25.3

(*a*) A metabolic alkalosis. Together with renal excretion of H^+ ions there will be excretion of potassium and retention of sodium.

(*b*) Pyloric stenosis with prolonged vomiting. Proportionately more H^+ ions than sodium or potassium are lost in the vomitus. Kidneys retain sodium preferentially to potassium or H^+ ions, enhancing the systemic alkalosis and maintaining an acidic urine.

Answer 25.4

(*a*) The left kidney is probably completely obstructed and the right partially. The most likely cause of bilateral asymmetric obstruction is a bladder tumour. The history of haematuria and the rapid decline in renal function make this diagnosis almost certain. Renal impairment following hypertension is usually found in the patient with accelerated hypertension, and is unusual and gradual in severe essential hypertension. A rapidly progressive glomerulonephritis could have been considered in the differential diagnosis before the IVP result was available.

(b) Cystoscopy is essential and showed in this patient an extensive bladder tumour. The left ureteric orifice could not be identified and the right was catheterized with difficulty. Injection of contrast demonstrated a hydro-ureter above the bladder.

(c) Virtually all middle-aged patients with haematuria require an IVP and cystoscopy regardless of their blood pressure.

Answer 25.5

Initial investigation must be directed towards treatable conditions including subacute combined degeneration of the spinal cord and syphilis. Blood and CSF serology should be checked and serum B_{12} concentrations. Diabetes can manifest similarly but would probably have been detected earlier. A lesion in the conus may only be found after myelography (and CT scanning at the time of the myelogram may be needed). The two remaining possibilities— Friedreich's ataxia and motor neurone disease—are both rare and untreatable.

Answer 25.6

(a) This woman had gout. The combination of a very painful joint with a raised serum urate makes this the most likely diagnosis.

(b) Gout should not be diagnosed (especially in a joint other than in the great toe) without aspiration of synovial fluid and examination under polarizing light to visualize the characteristic negatively birefringent crystals. In this case a primary bacterial arthritis would be diagnosed if the joint was not aspirated. Therapeutic confirmation could be obtained with colchicine therapy which will control the pain within hours.

(c) This attack of gout was precipitated by the thiazide diuretic taken to control the heart failure. All thiazide diuretics tend to decrease urinary urate excretion although the mechanism is unknown.

Answer 25.7

(*a*) From the information given the diagnosis was an obstructive jaundice and in a woman aged 62 years carcinoma of the pancreas is quite probable although gallstones could cause a similar picture.
(*b*) The coagulation deficiency is likely to be secondary to vitamin K malabsorption which is frequent in obstructive jaundice. This is due to a lack of bile salts which are essential for the emulsification and hence absorption of fats and the fat-soluble vitamins (A, D, K). In this patient two intramuscular doses of vitamin K resulted in a return to normal of the coagulation profile. The vitamin K-dependent clotting factors are II, VII, IX, X and the proteins C and S.

Answer 25.8

This woman had mixed connective tissue disease (MCTD). The history, high ESR and a positive ANF indicate an auto-immune state. The normal complement level excludes systemic lupus erythematosus. The speckled appearance of the ANF and the high titre of the antiribonuclear protein antibodies make the diagnosis.

MCTD usually has overlapping features of systemic lupus erythematosis, polymyositis, scleroderma and rheumatoid arthritis, and requires the presence of anti-ribonuclear proteins (RNP) to make the diagnosis.

Answer 25.9

(*a*) Partial gastrectomy.
(*b*) Iron deficiency anaemia and osteomalacia. There is failure of iron absorption because of reduced gastric acidity. The cause of vitamin D deficiency is less clear but may relate to a combination of dietary deficiency and failure of absorption. There is an increased risk of carcinoma developing in the gastric remnant.

Answer 25.10

(*a*) Diabetic ketoacidosis.
(*b*) Plasma lipid concentrations.
(*c*) Removal of lipid by ether extraction and reanalysis showed plasma sodium 130 mmol/l, potassium 5.0 mmol/l. The creatinine

is raised compared with the urea because of a combination of not eating and the presence of ketone bodies which react in the assay used for creatinine in most laboratories. Amylase concentrations are often raised substantially even when pancreatitis has not precipitated the diabetic ketoacidosis. A raised white cell count may be a sign of underlying infection (which may have triggered the ketoacidosis) but can occur in the absence of sepsis.

Answer 26.1

(a) This rhythm strip shows an atrial flutter with varying block—1:1 to 1:3. The 'saw-tooth' flutter waves obscure the isoelectric line.

(b) Underlying causes include ischaemic heart disease, hyperthyroidism and rheumatic heart disease. More rare causes are cardiomyopathy, acute febrile illnesses, pulmonary emboli, lone fibrillators (idiopathic) and pericarditis.

(c) The patient should be digitalized. This blocks A–V transmission of some of the atrial impulses, with slowing of the ventricular rate. In addition, the flutter may return to sinus rhythm and the digoxin may then be withdrawn.

Answer 26.2

(a) Falling asleep easily.

(b) Obesity—she weighed 141.5 kg.

(c) Pickwickian or fat boy syndrome. It is generally held that massive obesity impedes respiration, leading to hypoventilation and chronic hypoxia. It has also been suggested that a hypothalamic lesion could cause both hypoventilation and obesity. Clinical tests of lung function and chest X-rays are normal.

Answer 26.3

(a) A pituitary chromophobe or basophil adenoma producing an excess of ACTH.

(b) He will be deeply pigmented—Nelson's syndrome. Adrenalectomy removes the site of excess cortisol production but not the primary cause. The pituitary continues to produce an excess of ACTH (normal range about 15–80 pg/ml) and β-MSH—the β-MSH excess leads to excess pigmentation.

(c) Bitemporal hemianopia occurs due to compression of the optic chiasm by the upward expansion of the pituitary tumour first compressing the decussating fibres.

(d) Treatment would probably involve surgical removal of the tumour and possibly radiotherapy.

Answer 26.4

(a) A CT scan may help to elucidate the nature of the left renal mass and arteriography may then be indicated.

(b) This man had a hypernephroma as suggested by the haematuria and the abnormal IVP. Raised alkaline phosphatase is occasionally associated with a hypernephroma in the absence of metastatic spread—this is unexplained. Liver function returns to normal after removal of the renal cancer. Arteriography produces a characteristic appearance and should be bilateral so that small contralateral tumours are not missed.

Answer 26.5

(a) The high CSF protein, mixed cellular response and low glucose in an illness developing over 10 days are suggestive of tuberculous meningitis. High CSF protein and low glucose concentrations are only infrequently found in viral meningitis and the cellular response is typically predominantly lymphocytic. The onset of viral and of bacterial meningitis is much more rapid than in this example.

(b) There are three other investigations needed: Ziehl–Neelsen staining of the CSF, the setting up of Loewenstein–Jensen cultures and a chest X-ray. In an adult, cytological examination of the CSF is necessary because carcinomatous meningitis has a chronic deteriorating course together with a mixed pleocytosis and reduction in the CSF glucose.

Answer 26.6

The clue to this question is that the blood was obtained with 'some difficulty'. The figures show respiratory alkalosis but this may have

214

been induced via hyperventilation because of pain at the time of arterial puncture. Unless the patient has cause for a respiratory alkalosis the blood gas data should be interpreted with care.

Answer 26.7

(a) This infant had haemorrhagic disease of the newborn as shown by the normal coagulation indices with the exception of a prolonged prothrombin time. Other sites of bleeding include the gastrointestinal tract and the skin. The lesion is common in low birth weight babies.

(b) The treatment is intramuscular vitamin K which corrects the prolonged prothrombin time within a few hours. Occasionally a transfusion may be needed.

The present practice of giving vitamin K to all babies at birth, particularly those of low weight and of instrumental delivery, makes the condition now relatively unusual.

Answer 26.8

This patient had a subnormal response to synthetic ACTH. This is very suggestive of therapeutically induced adrenal insufficiency secondary to prednisolone given to the patient during the survival of the transplanted kidney. A normal response to intramuscular synthetic ACTH is an increment in the 30 minute serum cortisol of at least 190 nmol/l (about 7 µg/100 ml) with the serum cortisol rising to at least 500 nmol/l (about 20 µg/100 ml).

Answer 26.9

(a) This woman had gradually become digoxin intoxicated as indicated by the plasma digoxin of 2.7 ng/ml, and the rapid pulse was shown to be due to a mixture of atrial fibrillation and ventricular ectopic beats. Generally, patients with plasma digoxin levels above 2.5 ng/ml are considered to be toxic but clinical toxicity may occur at lower doses and is enhanced by hypokalaemia or hypercalcaemia.

(b) Renal function judged by blood urea and plasma creatinine appear superficially to be normal. About 35% of total body digoxin is excreted daily and its excretion is approximately proportional to creatinine clearance. However, for either blood urea or plasma creatinine to rise, the GFR has to be reduced by about 50% and sometimes more if the muscle mass is reduced and protein intake poor, as in many elderly people. Hence, in this woman, despite apparently normal renal function, the GFR had gradually fallen (due to senile nephron loss and perhaps renal emboli from the left atrium) and her dose of digoxin slowly became inappropriately high. It was found subsequently that 0.0625 mg of digoxin daily was adequate.

Answer 26.10

(a) This patient had a macrocytic anaemia in the presence of a normal serum B_{12} concentration. Some severely psoriatic patients need methotrexate to control their skin condition. Methotrexate binds to dihydrofolate reductase, thereby blocking folate metabolism and producing macrocytic anaemia.
(b) The anaemia must be treated with folinic acid and not by folic acid (pteroylglutamic acid). Folinic acid is already reduced and is beyond the metabolic step blocked by folic acid antagonists.
(c) Up to 50% of patients taking methotrexate for psoriasis develop hepatic fibrosis and this can progress to cirrhosis. This can be minimized by giving large once-weekly doses rather than smaller daily doses.

Answer 27.1

This rhythm strip shows a 2:1 heart block (sino-atrial block). The ventricular rate is 48 and the atrial rate 96 per minute.

Answer 27.2

(a) The blood gas tensions fit an acute exacerbation of chronic bronchitis but the pH is very low and bicarbonate is too low for a respiratory acidosis. The figures are those of both respiratory and non-respiratory acidosis.

(*b*) The patient required urgent investigation for causes of non-respiratory acidosis. Blood glucose: diabetic ketoacidosis; salicylate poisoning; lactate concentration; shock or poisoning by biguanides, methanol or ethanol. He had taken an overdose of aspirin tablets as his chest condition was deteriorating.

Answer 27.3

(*a*) The child was very small for her age. There was evidence of malabsorption from the xylose test and the low serum albumin. The calcium corrects into the normal range: corrected calcium = calcium + $[(46 - \text{albumin}) \times 0.02]$, in this case $2.00 + [(46 - 28) \times 0.02] = 2.36$ mmol/l. The peak D-xylose concentration should be >30 mg/100 ml and normally >22% of a 5 g load (or >17% of a 25 g load) appears in the urine in the 5 hours after ingestion. Xylose absorption is normal in pancreatic malabsorption.

(*b*) If renal function is poor or there is a large amount of peripheral oedema then the xylose absorption test is unreliable.

(*c*) A sweat test and jejunal biopsy are necessary to diagnose cystic fibrosis and coeliac disease respectively. The presence of reducing substances in the stools would be evidence of sugar malabsorption and specific sugar tolerance tests could be undertaken to elucidate that aspect.

Answer 27.4

This patient had a systemic acidosis with acid urine, hypocalciuria and one of the histological features of osteomalacia. The mean width of osteoid borders in undecalcified normal bone is about 9 μm. The urine is acid which is almost invariable in chronic renal failure and contrasts with a renal tubular acidosis in which the urine rarely has a pH of below 6.

The differential diagnosis includes renal calcification secondary to hypercalcaemia, renal cortical necrosis or longstanding renal tuberculosis. The first of these conditions is the most common in Britain. The low urine calcium is explained by the renal failure—when the GFR falls to below 20–25 ml/min, hypocalciuria (less than 2.5 mmol/day (100 mg/day)) is virtually constant regardless of the concentration of the serum calcium.

Answer 27.5

(a) Bacterial meningitis. There is a neutrophil leucocytosis in the CSF with a raised protein concentration and a reduced glucose relative to the blood glucose.

(b) Gram staining of the CSF is essential. When the white count is as high as this the CSF would be visibly turbid as it was collected.

(c) Intravenous benzyl penicillin and chloramphenicol remain the standard treatment of meningitis in this age group when the causative organism is unknown.

(d) Leucocyte metabolism utilizes the glucose in the CSF (not the bacteria)!

(e) The immediate immunoglobulin response is IgM.

Answer 27.6

(a) This woman had osteoporosis as shown by the normal serum calcium and phosphate and the normal urinary calcium. The raised alkaline phosphatase in this patient was a reflection of the fracture and fell to normal when the bone healed.

(b) Confirmation of the diagnosis usually rests upon radiological thinning and reduction in the trabecular pattern of bones, the femoral necks and vertebrae being the best areas to show these features. Bone densitometry and bone biopsy may also be used.

(c) Osteoporosis may be secondary to (i) natural ageing; (ii) prolonged immobilization (either local or generalized); (iii) partial gastrectomy; (iv) other causes of malabsorption; (v) Cushing's syndrome; (vi) hyperthyroidism; (vii) liver disease; (viii) hypogonadism; (ix) scurvy; (x) diabetes; (xi) long-term exposure to heparin (e.g. in patients on maintenance haemodialysis).

Answer 27.7

(a) This woman had Addisonian megaloblastic anaemia (pernicious anaemia, PA).

(b) The diagnosis should be proved by finding a low vitamin B_{12} concentration (less than 100 ng/l) (100 pg/ml), a histamine-fast achlorhydria and defective radio-vitamin B_{12} absorption (Schilling test). In practice achlorhydria is not usually sought, but antibodies to intrinsic factor (IF) are looked for. Note that a bone marrow biopsy does not prove the diagnosis as it will only show non-specific megaloblastic changes.

(c) Anti-IF antibodies occur in 50% of patients and are of two types: type I ('blocking') bind the intrinsic factor B_{12} binding site and type II bind the ileal binding site. Anti-gastric parietal cell antibodies are found in 85–90% of patients but are a non-specific finding. In addition, auto-antibodies to other organs are frequently present—especially against the components of the thyroid glands.

Answer 27.8

(a) The chromatin-positive buccal smear indicates the presence of two X chromosomes in a cell, i.e. a genotypic female. Only one X is active; the other is seen as a darkly staining spot at the periphery of the nucleus, the Barr body. In the case of a genotypic male, no Barr body is seen and the patient is chromatin negative.

The urinary ketosteroid excretion was within the normal range.

(b) (i) Pseudohermaphroditism. In female pseudohermaphroditism the clitoris may be enlarged by exogenous steroids (progesterones given to the mother in the treatment of threatened abortion) or endogenous steroids in the adrenogenital syndrome, in which the urinary excretion of ketosteroids would be raised. In male pseudohermaphroditism, by contrast, the gonads are testes, the karyotype is 46XY, but the external genitalia are intermediate and look basically female.

(ii) True hermaphroditism. The patient has both ovary and testis. The karyotype may be either male or female, chromatin positive or negative. Mosaicism has been described. Gonads may be palpable in the inguinal region or the labia.

(iii) Hypospadias with a bifid scrotum would be in the clinical differential diagnosis but buccal smear and karyotype exclude it in this example.

(iv) Simple labial fusion may occur in the female.

(c) If the gonads were palpable in the perineum, gonadal biopsy would be indicated together with laparoscopy to define the pelvic anatomy.

Answer 27.9

This echocardiogram shows an atrial myxoma in the mitral 'funnel'. Compare the mitral area of *Figure 27.1* with the mitral

219

area of *Figure 31.2*. An atrial myxoma is rare but produces a characteristic echocardiogram, as do mitral stenosis and pericardial effusion.

Answer 27.10

(*a*) This girl had acute on chronic renal failure as shown by the high urea, the haemoconcentration and low urine volume accompanied by low urinary osmolarity.

Patients with chronic renal failure being followed regularly in Outpatients are usually started on maintenance dialysis treatment when the urea is 50 mmol/l or less.

(*b*) Immediate management involves insertion of a central venous pressure line and administration of large quantities of normal saline until the central venous pressure has been returned to normal.

(*c*) It is very probable that tetracycline had been prescribed for acne. This drug, if given to patients in renal failure, produces a brisk rise in blood urea with rapid clinical deterioration.

Answer 28.1

There are no P waves, the QRS complexes are broadened and are merging with the T waves. All are features of hyperkalaemia. The plasma potassium was 8.3 mmol/l (mEq/l) in this man.

Answer 28.2

(*a*) This man should be considered to have *Pneumocystis carinii* infection and treated as such without delay.

(*b*) The patient should be bronchoscoped and brushings and washings taken which might demonstrate the parasite. A transbronchial lung biopsy should be performed and can be touch-imprinted on to microscope slides and stained with Gomorri's methenamine silver nitrate to demonstrate the organism. Sputum should also be examined for tubercle bacilli.

(*c*) Regardless of the bronchoscopic findings the patient should receive pentamidine or co-trimoxazole or both. Withdrawal of immunosuppressive therapy may be necessary. *P. carinii* infection has a high mortality and it is better to lose the transplant kidney and save the patient than to lose both.

Answer 28.3

(*a*) If the mother's blood group is O rhesus positive then ABO incompatibility would be likely. The baby had unconjugated hyperbilirubinaemia without significant anaemia and normal liver cell function. The Coombs' test is usually negative and detection of abnormal anti-A in the mother is not always possible.

(*b*) Breast milk jaundice should be considered and evidence of infection should be sought, especially if the baby appears unwell; among the investigations the urine must be cultured. If the jaundice were to persist, hypothyroidism or galactosaemia should be considered.

(*c*) Treatment includes adequate fluid intake, temporary withdrawal of breast milk and phototherapy until a sustained fall in bilirubin is achieved.

Answer 28.4

(*a*) The presumptive diagnosis is that of an acute transplant rejection as indicated by the high neutrophil count with the reduced lymphocyte count and the low urine volume. In addition, flu-like symptoms are frequently associated with acute graft rejection. The development of proteinuria or an increase if already present are features of transplant rejection, as are reduced urine volumes and creatinine clearance when compared with previous measurements.

(*b*) Other findings include fever, hypertension, tenderness of the transplanted kidney, increase in urinary lymphocytes, fall in circulating platelets and serum complement components.

Answer 28.5

(*a*) This woman had the Ramsay Hunt syndrome (herpes zoster of the geniculate ganglion). Although the majority of patients make some recovery, this is complete in only 50%.

(*b*) Involvement of the fifth cranial nerve can lead to sensory loss over the face, and of the ninth nerve, to numbness of the palate. The vagus is the motor nerve of the palate.

(*c*) Investigations to exclude myeloma are needed in view of the very high ESR, the rouleaux on the blood film and the hypergammaglobulinaemia. Skull, vertebrae and pelvis should be X-rayed, urine tested for Bence-Jones proteinuria and the bone marrow examined.

Answer 28.6

(a) The infant has galactosaemia (deficiency of galactose-1-phosphate uridyltransferase); reducing substance which was not glucose was present in the urine.

(b) The diagnosis is confirmed by measurement of red cell galactose-1-phosphate uridyltransferase.

(c) The child should be given a lactose-free diet—that is, the use of lactose-free infant formula.

(d) The parents should be told that the condition is an autosomal recessive (occurring in approximately 1 in 60 000 births); there is therefore a 1 in 4 chance of an affected individual from each pregnancy. Antenatal diagnosis is possible.

Answer 28.7

A high platelet count of this degree may be found in the following:

(i) Chronic blood loss.
(ii) Post-splenectomy.
(iii) Polycythaemia rubra vera.
(iv) Myelosclerosis.
(v) Haemorrhagic thrombocythaemia. In this rare condition the platelets are morphologically abnormal and functionally defective. The spleen is often atrophic or absent.

Answer 28.8

(a) The clinical features might suggest Klinefelter's syndrome—but these patients have primary hypogonadism with decreased plasma concentration of testosterone (normal range 9–24 nmol/l). The increased prolactin concentration (normal range less than 10 μg/l in adult males) with the depressed plasma testosterone suggests a hypothalamic lesion.

(*b*) This man would therefore need:

    (*i*)   visual field testing;
    (*ii*) further endocrine assessment of the hypothalamic–pituitary axis;
    (*iii*) X-rays of the sella turcica—coned simple X-rays and CT scan.

He was shown to have a pituitary tumour, extending upwards, compressing the hypothalamus and leading to hyperprolactinaemia.

Answer 28.9

(*a*) A heart transplant.

(*b*) Such hearts lack innervation, as shown by the high resting heart rate (no vagal tone). The slow response to exercise is thought to be mediated by circulating catecholamines. The increase in the left ventricular end diastolic pressure and cardiac output upon increasing venous return is a demonstration of the Frank–Starling mechanism—the force of contraction is proportional to stretching the heart muscle.

Answer 28.10

(*a*) This woman had accelerated (malignant) hypertension. The normal urine microscopy and IVP virtually exclude primary renal disease. High concentrations of circulating renin are usually found in accelerated hypertension and are thought to be a reflection of renal damage secondary to the high pressure rather than a primary phenomenon.

(*b*) The increase in plasma renin is to be expected: frusemide causes renin release secondary to the sodium depletion it produces. Diazoxide causes renin release as a result of the increase in circulating volume consequent upon the peripheral vascular dilatation it produces. A fall in GFR after aggressive hypotensive therapy is also to be expected; with stabilization of the blood pressure the GFR usually returns to, or may rise above, the pretreatment level.

(*c*) Diazoxide is a very potent hypotensive drug but has two important side-effects: intense sodium retention and a diabetogenic action. All patients taking diazoxide should receive a potent 'loop' diuretic.

Answer 29.1

(*a*) This trace shows a wandering pacemaker. The ventricular rate is constant but the P waves vary, becoming biphasic and inverted with shortening of the PR interval. The term 'wandering pacemaker' is considered by some to be a misnomer as the rhythm is dual, both sino-atrial (SA) and arteriovenous (AV) nodes discharging spontaneously with variable asynchronism.

(*b*) This condition may be found by chance in healthy individuals but is also associated with digoxin therapy. In the latter circumstance the dose should be reduced.

Answer 29.2

(*a*) This woman has Conn's syndrome (primary hyperaldosteronism). This may either be an aldosterone-producing adenoma or carcinoma, idiopathic hyperaldosteronism or glucocorticoid-remediable hyperaldosteronism. Increased urinary and plasma aldosterone concentrations are found, and hyporeninaemia. This results in hypokalaemic alkalosis, sodium retention and hypertension.

(*b*) Hypokalaemia can cause muscle weakness and cramps. In the kidney it causes local prostaglandin synthesis which antagonizes the effect of the antidiuretic hormone (ADH) on the distal nephron. This results in polyuria and, combined with a plasma sodium which is usually at the upper limit of normal, results in thirst and polydipsia.

Answer 29.3

She may have malabsorption due to coeliac disease, sensitivity to cow's milk or infestation (for example with *Giardia lamblia*). Her diet may be generally poor and specifically deficient in vitamin D. Because of her ethnic background she may get little exposure to sunlight, leading to reduced vitamin D synthesis. Chappatis may cause malabsorption of calcium because of their high phytate content which forms insoluble complexes in the gut lumen.

Answer 29.4

She is alkalotic, hypocapnic and has a normal Po_2. The blood glucose was 12 mmol/l. She is hyperventilating and was deliberately trying to avoid dialysing for the necessary amount of time. The natural response of nursing staff to a patient becoming short of breath during dialysis is to stop dialysis, particularly when the patient suggests that it is exacerbating her symptoms—as in this case. This woman had many social problems which resulted in manipulative behaviour and her being on a type of renal replacement therapy which is not ideal for insulin-dependent diabetics with end-stage renal failure.

Answer 29.5

(*a*) The phenytoin level is below the therapeutic range (usually 3–16 mg/l) while the phenobarbitone concentration is modestly elevated (therapeutic range 4.0–4.2 mg/l). Two factors may account for the phenytoin levels: the patient may not be taking the dose prescribed or the dosage may not have been increased relative to the child's weight, if he has been on the drug over a number of years.

(*b*) The phenobarbitone level may be associated with hyperactivity and distractedness.

Answer 29.6

(*a*) This patient had an uncompensated respiratory alkalosis consequent upon tachypnoea with wash-out of carbon dioxide.

(*b*) This was due to direct stimulation of the respiratory centre by salicylates. Renal excretion of bicarbonate will bring the pH back towards normal, producing a compensated respiratory alkalosis.

(*c*) Subsequently (in the absence of treatment) a combined respiratory and metabolic acidosis develops due to the following:

(*i*) Increasing concentration of salicylate depresses the respiratory centre and induces carbon dioxide retention (respiratory acidosis).

(*ii*) Renal function becomes impaired because of hypotension and dehydration with retention of organic metabolic acids.

(*iii*) Salicylates impair carbohydrate metabolism with accumulation of acetoacetate, lactic and pyruvic acid.

(*iv*) Salicylate and its metabolites are acidic and further enhance the metabolic acidosis.

Answer 29.7

(*a*) It is unlikely that this child had leukaemia despite white blood cell precursors in the blood film as the platelet count was normal, there was an elevated reticulocyte count and marked abnormalities of the red blood cells—hypochromia, microchromia, poikilocytosis and target cells. This is a leuco-erythroblastic blood picture but the major abnormality lies within the erythrocytes. This child had thalassaemia major in which abnormal peripheral white blood cells are found. The red blood cell findings in this case are characteristic and one would expect the haemoglobin to be in the region of 5–7 g/dl (g/100 ml) with a target cell count of 10–30% and a red cell count of $2–3 \times 10^{12}/l$ ($2–3 \times 10^6/mm^3$).

(*b*) Children with thalassaemia major fail to thrive, are pale with enlarged spleen and liver and have 'mongoloid' facies.

(*c*) Haemoglobin electrophoresis would show various degrees of increased HbF and low or raised HbA_2. HbA may be absent.

(*d*) (*i*) The skull shows thickened diploë with thin outer and inner tables with perpendicular striae appearing between the tables leading to the 'hair-on-end' appearance.

(*ii*) In long bones, especially the distal ends of the femora, the medulla is increased and the cortex thinned. Short bones tend to be rectangular in contour with a trabeculated medulla giving a mosaic pattern.

Answer 29.8

(*a*) The macrocytosis (MCV of 115 fl (μm^3)) coupled with diarrhoea and the appearances of the jejunal biopsy indicate a probable malabsorptive condition.

(*b*) The normal jejunal plasma cell population consists of mainly IgA-synthesizing cells and a change to IgM predominance is seen in coeliac disease. In addition, in this condition serum IgM is decreased in about 60% of patients and there appears to be a higher incidence of isolated IgA deficiency. Antireticulin antibodies may be demonstrated also in coeliac disease.

(c) There is an increased incidence of HLA B1 and B8 antigen in coeliac patients compared with control populations.

Answer 29.9

(a) Right ventricular cardiomyopathy (Uhl's anomaly or arrhythmogenic right ventricular dysplasia or parchment heart) causes sudden death during strenuous exercise in young people.

(b) Other causes of sudden death are aortic stenosis, myocarditis, congenital coronary artery anomalies, premature coronary artery disease and syndromes involving prolonged QT intervals.

(c) There is partial or complete absence of the right ventricular myocardium which is replaced by fibrous or adipose tissue. This may be so complete in some cases that the appearances are of paper with virtual apposition of endocardium and epicardium.

Answer 29.10

(a) Multiple endocrine neoplasia type 2a (MEN 2a or Sipple's syndrome); a parathyroid adenoma (raised calcium), a medullary carcinoma of the thyroid (MCT) (normal T_3 and TSH with a mass in the neck) and a phaeochromocytoma (hypertension).

(b) A provocation test of calcitonin secretion should be performed. In cases of MCT, the concentrations rise dramatically in response to an infusion of calcium or pentagastrin or ingestion of alcohol even if basal concentrations are normal. Plasma and urinary catecholamines should be measured to confirm the diagnosis of phaeochromocytoma.

(c) Inheritance is autosomal dominant (AD) and the defect is on the short arm of chromosome 1. When cases are identified, all first- and second-degree relatives should be screened by means of calcitonin secretion provocation tests, as above.

Answer 30.1

(a) This patient had a VSD with a right-to-left shunt. If pulmonary hypertension is present this is known as Eisenmenger's syndrome. There is a step down in oxygen saturation between the left atrium and the left ventricle. There is therefore venous mixing in the left ventricle—the venous blood coming from the right ventricle. The shunt in a VSD is at first left to right. Pulmonary hypertension may develop and right ventricular pressure rises above left ventricular pressure so the shunt reverses to right to left. (b) Surgery is contra-indicated because of the right-to-left shunt. If the VSD were repaired it would be followed by right ventricular failure which might be fatal.

Answer 30.2

(a) This woman had hypercalcaemia, hypermagnesaemia with a low serum phosphate and hypercalciuria. The simplest explanation of these findings is primary hyperparathyroidism complicated by (i) the development of a duodenal ulcer which had led to the development of an iron deficiency anaemia; (ii) the development of a renal stone which had led to an *Escherichia coli* urinary tract infection and haematuria. The elevated calcium and depressed phosphate are characteristic of primary hyperparathyroidism. Hypermagnesaemia is found in a proportion of these patients and returns to normal with removal of the parathyroid adenoma.

(b) Radiologically an IVP and barium meal are indicated and in that order so that no barium remains in the gut to obscure X-rays of the renal tract.

(c) The primary abnormality can be confirmed by measurement of circulating parathyroid hormone (PTH) concentration although from the above data it would not be necessary.

Answer 30.3

(a) Hypocalcaemia is the probable cause of the convulsion. In practice such a baby would probably be bottle fed and the phosphate load from the cow's milk formula might well depress the ionized calcium although the total calcium quoted in this example is not particularly low. Hypocalcaemic convulsions do not occur in the breast-fed baby and do not arise in the bottle-fed until the baby has been receiving milk for several days. Hypoglycaemia is a significant and treatable cause of convulsions in a low birth weight baby as quoted but a blood glucose concentration of 1.7 mmol/l (30 mg/100 ml) is not of the order to be symptomatic and the child would probably present earlier.

(*b*) A lumbar puncture would be a necessary investigation—neonatal meningitis must be excluded. Intracranial bleeding in association with haemorrhagic disease of the newborn and/or perinatal asphyxia are possibilities.

Answer 30.4

(*a*) The biochemical constitution of any stone or fragment of gravel passed *per urethra* should be determined. The urine cyanide–nitroprusside test should be performed (positive in the presence of cystinuria, homocystinuria and Fanconi's syndrome). Urine amino acid chromatography is the definitive test.

(*b*) He has cystinuria. Cystine, ornithine, arginine and lysine were found on urine amino acid chromatography and the cyanide–nitroprusside test was positive. (The reagents are toxic and this test is rarely performed now.) Cystinuria is an autosomal recessive condition and the hexagonal crystals are characteristic. Treatment consists of high oral fluid intake night and day (4 litres per 24 h) and alkalinization of the urine with oral sodium bicarbonate (to maintain a urinary pH of >8). Some patients require oral D-penicillamine which reacts with cystine to produce a more soluble complex that does not precipitate.

Answer 30.5

(*a*) This man had Paget's disease (osteitis deformans) of the pubic rami and acetabula. Also, as is common when bone close to large joints becomes pagetoid, osteoarthritis developed which contributed to the pain.

(*b*) The raised serum alkaline phosphatase and urinary hydroxyproline excretion reflect osteoblastic and osteoclastic activity respectively.

(*c*) If symptoms cannot be controlled with analgesics and non-steroidal anti-inflammatory drugs, a number of different agents are available: they include fluoride, glucagon, mithramycin, calcitonin and diphosphonates. The last two are the most practical therapeutic agents. Either of these drugs will reduce elevated serum alkaline phosphatase and the urinary excretion of hydroxyproline.

Answer 30.6

This is an example of interaction between clofibrate and warfarin. Both are protein bound and, as some of the binding sites for warfarin were already occupied by clofibrate, disproportionately severe anticoagulation occurred. The prothrombin time was found to be 75 seconds with a control of 15 seconds although the doses of warfarin given were correct in proportion to the weight of the patient.

Answer 30.7

(a) This man had an obstructive jaundice and Coombs' negative spherocytosis. The combination suggests a long-continued haemolytic anaemia with the development of bile pigment gallstones. Bilirubin is present in the urine because of the obstructive jaundice. Spherocytes cannot be biconcave and have a normal volume; hence their diameter is less than normal. Osmotic fragility is increased.

(b) This man should be questioned regarding his antecedents. Hereditary (congenital) spherocytosis is an autosomal dominant and other members of his family would have had the condition. However, this condition could arise as a mutation in the absence of a positive family history.

(c) The spleen was palpable.

Answer 30.8

(a) This boy had developed graft-versus-host disease (GVHD). The aetiology is obscure. The skin changes may be acute at 7–21 days after the transplant, or later within the first 6 weeks, with a diffuse reddening and scaling, lichenoid lesions or bullae. Liver dysfunction may be severe and fatal.

(b) T-cell depletion of donor marrow is now routinely undertaken using combinations of physicochemical separation, binding to plant lectins and monoclonal anti-T-cell antibodies. This patient could have had cytomegalovirus infection (CMV), and CMV vaccination or hyperimmune gamma-globulin infusions may help to reduce this serious complication.